THE RELATIONAL TRAUMA OF INCEST

The Relational Trauma of Incest

A *Family-Based Approach to Treatment*

Marcia Sheinberg
Peter Fraenkel

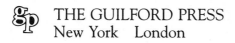

THE GUILFORD PRESS
New York   London

©2001 The Guilford Press
A Division of Guilford Publications, Inc.
72 Spring Street, New York, NY 10012
www.guilford.com

Printed in the United States of America

This book is printed on acid-free paper.

Last digit is print number: 9 8 7 6 5 4 3 2 1

Library of Congress Cataloging-in-Publication Data

Sheinberg, Marcia.
      The relational trauma of incest: a family-based approach to treatment /
   Marcia Sheinberg, Peter Fraenkel.
          p. cm.
   Includes bibliographical references and index.
   ISBN 1-57230-599-1
        1. Incest—Treatment   2. Incest victims—Rehabilitation. 3. Psychotherapy.
   4. Family psychotherapy.   I. Fraenkel, Peter.   II. Title.
   RC560.I53 S543 2000
   616.85'8360651—dc21

00-061766

About the Authors

Marcia Sheinberg, MSW, is the Director of Training and Clinical Services at the Ackerman Institute for the Family. She is a cofounder of its Gender and Violence Project and the founder and Director of the Incest Project. An advisory editor for *Family Process* and a member of the editorial board of the *Journal of Feminist Family Therapy*, she has published widely in professional journals on the treatment of chronic illness in the family, the role of gender in relationships, the treatment of obsessional disorders, domestic violence, larger systems, incest, and clinical innovations in couple and family therapy. In addition, she maintains an active private practice in which she treats and consults with individuals, couples, and families on a variety of clinical issues.

Peter Fraenkel, PhD, is Associate Professor of Psychology in the Doctoral Program in Clinical Psychology at The City College of the City University of New York. At the Ackerman Institute for the Family, he is a member of the Teaching Faculty, Director of Research and Clinical Member in the Incest Project, and Director of the Center for Time, Work, and the Family. Dr. Fraenkel is also Clinical Assistant Professor of Psychiatry at New York University Medical School and Director of the Prevention and Relationship Enhancement Program in the NYU Child Study Center. Dr. Fraenkel has published and lectured extensively in the areas of family systems theory and integration, incest, families and time, welfare to work, and distress prevention programs for couples and families. He is an ad hoc editor for *Family Process* and advisory editor for the *Journal of Marital and Family Therapy*. He is also in private practice.

Both Ms. Sheinberg and Dr. Fraenkel are internationally recognized and regularly present in Asia, Europe, Latin America, the United States, and Canada.

Acknowledgments

We wish to thank our colleagues from the New York agencies who over the years have worked with us on the Incest Project: Jon Frankel, Carmen Goris, Libbe Madsen, Manuel Muñoz, and Ann Richmond. We also thank the directors of the agencies and programs for their joint vision of a coordinated system of service for abused children and their families: Jane A. Barker, Ruth Rosen Cohen, Tony Cucchiari, Paul Gitelson, Lucy N. Friedman, Phil Hayden, Jaime Inclan, Antonio Pagan, Alan B. Siskind, Peter Steinglass, Carol Stokinger, and Lewis Zuckman. We also wish to acknowledge our colleagues at the Ackerman Institute for the Family who have at different times participated in the Incest Project: Judy Stern Peck (who codirected the consortium of participating agencies), Ray DeMaio, Paul Feinberg, Sonja Rolovic, Sippio Small, and Gillian Walker. Marcia Scanlon was indispensable as administrative assistant to the Project. We appreciate Abbe Steinglass's creative work in developing an art program to supplement the clinical work. We remain extremely grateful to Arthur Maslow for his early encouragement and support.

We could not have done this work without our colleague Fiona True, our clinical partner from the inception of the Project to the present. She is the therapist in a number of the case examples included in this book. In addition, through spearheading many of our community-based trainings, she brought the relational approach to a variety of institutional settings.

Finally, the clinical work, training activities, and research were made possible by the generous support of numerous anonymous donors as well as several foundations—specifically, the Frances L. and Edwin L. Cummings Memorial Fund, the Educational Foundation of America, the Ittleson Foundation, the Ms. Foundation, the Lucy and Henry Moses Foundation, the New Land Foundation, the Ronald McDonald Children's Charities of New York, and the Donald and Shelly Rubin Foundation.

We are deeply appreciative to Virginia Goldner for her thoughtful comments on an earlier draft of this book, and to Ellen Wachtel for her careful reading and detailed comments on various chapters.

We have been blessed with not one, but two, outstanding editors at The Guilford Press. We started with Kitty Moore, whose talent for discerning the core ideas helped us bring these into bas-relief, and whose combination of patience and prodding kept the book moving along even when many other professional and life commitments interfered. Jim Nageotte came on board at the critical end phase. His insightful comments and useful distinctions were essential as we tied together all the loose ends.

Finally, we cannot adequately express the appreciation we feel toward the families who let us into their lives and taught us what appears in the following pages.

Preface

A hallmark of the experience of incest is the maelstrom of intense confusion and contradiction felt by children and their families. The acts of the offending family member shake the very foundations of family relationships—relationships that at their best are built upon care and trust. Abused children and other nonoffending family members often feel torn between love and hate, self-blame versus blame of the offending member, the wish to restore family unity versus the need to prevent further abuse, and the desire to go on as if nothing happened versus the need to face the awful truth. As a result, abused children and their families are often left not knowing what to do next, what to believe, how to think about themselves and each other, and how to feel. These painful confusions can immobilize them and make it quite difficult to move beyond the abuse safely. Although not all incestuously abused children experience clinical levels of posttraumatic symptomatology or other psychological and behavioral disturbance, virtually all abused children and other nonoffending family members experience what we call *relational trauma*—disruption in the sense of trustworthiness, openness, and clarity of family relationships, and the emotional turmoil, loyalty binds, and dilemmas that result. This relational trauma is found in both the negative effects on interactions among family members and in the child's internal representations of family relationships and him- or herself.

Recognition of the inevitability and power of the relational trauma associated with incest led to the development of the relational approach to treatment described in this book. In essence, this "relational approach"[1] focuses on strengthening the healing potential of family relationships. Beginning in 1990, this approach was developed in a clinical project on incest at the Ackerman Institute for the Family, which initially leaned on ideas Marcia Sheinberg and her colleagues developed earlier in an Institute project on domestic violence. One of the key insights that emerged from the Domestic Violence Project was that in order for women to become truly able to protect themselves from further abuse, they needed the opportunity to honor and give voice to their complex feelings and attachments toward their violent partners—not only their fear and anger, but also their love and concern (Goldner, Penn, Sheinberg, & Walker, 1990). Another critical insight from the work of this group was that a clear moral perspective on violence—with the violent partner viewed as solely and completely responsible for these acts no matter how provocative the woman—could exist within a therapy that also looked at problem patterns to which both partners contributed. In other words, productive and safety-engendering work in this area required the therapist to live with the tension of holding a linear causal view of violence while simultaneously adopting a circular causal view of the relationship problems surrounding the violence. The Domestic Violence Project also actively engaged the problem of domestic violence as not only a therapeutic issue but also an example of work at the boundary between therapy and institutions of social control such as the police and the courts.

As the Incest Project clinicians began to see families in our clinic—many of whom were poor and living in the inner city—it quickly became apparent that abuse and the events surrounding disclosure constituted an extremely powerful stigmatizing and disempowering experience in the lives of poor children and women. The reports of these families made clear the often traumatizing impact of their contact with those professionals and agencies appointed to serve their needs for assessment, protection, and

---

[1]Our use of the term "relational approach" developed independently of the Stone Center's use of this term (cf. Bergman & Surrey, 1994; Jordan, Kaplan, Miller, Stiver, & Surrey, 1991) and is also to be distinguished from the relational perspective in psychoanalysis (Greenberg & Mitchell, 1983). For the Stone Center writers, the term "relational" primarily forms a conceptual bridge from psychoanalytic to interpersonal or contextual conceptions of self, and for relational theory in psychoanalysis, the bridge is between the object relations and interpersonal analytic school. For us, the term "relational" primarily has utility in providing a bridge or point of commonality among the three contextual theories that inform our approach: systems, social constructionist, and feminist.

treatment—the so-called "secondary victimization" (Levitt, Owen, & Truchsess, 1991), "secondary trauma," or "system-induced" trauma (Conte, 1984). Poor families are more likely to experience secondary trauma than are more economically advantaged families because poor families are more likely to have the abuse reported to child protective services (CPS) and to have the disclosure and treatment handled through public agencies (Knutson, 1995). Marcia recognized the need not only to work with families in therapy, but also to work to transform the larger system so that families' "treatment"—in the broad sense of the word—will be humane and consistent in all their contacts with professionals.

In that spirit, Marcia formed a consortium of agencies in New York City that work with sexually abused children—including social service, legal, medical, and therapy services—and developed procedures to coordinate services among these agencies (Peck, Sheinberg, & Akamatsu, 1995; Sheinberg, 1992). Both within and outside the consortium of agencies, we also began to conduct training programs for front-line professionals. Fiona True, our close colleague since the beginning of this work, took the lead in providing this community-based training.

In order to facilitate this training, Peter Fraenkel, who joined the Ackerman Incest Project in 1992 as both a clinical member and director of research, took the lead in writing a detailed handbook for these professionals (Fraenkel, Sheinberg, & True, 1996). In bringing an interest in the broader conceptual issues surrounding psychotherapy integration (Fraenkel, 1994, 1995, 1997; Fraenkel & Pinsof, 2000), he contributed to extending and refining the theoretical ideas underlying the approach. He also brought a "research lens" to the program, both in evaluating the success of the community-based training and in conducting qualitative research on families' experiences in the therapy (Fraenkel et al., 1998). The research fit with the Incest Project's commitment to working collaboratively with families, as family members' weekly reports of their therapy experiences influenced the continuing evolution of the therapy approach.

WHY WE WROTE THIS BOOK

Over the past decade or so, there has been an explosion of literature and resources on virtually every aspect of child sexual abuse and its treatment. In the face of the burgeoning literature, why would we write a book about our approach to treatment of families in which there has been incest? The first reason is that the rates of abuse appear to be increasing; thus, more treatment will be needed, and more clinicians than ever before will encounter families in which there has been incest. Second, a number of recent research findings support the need for a treatment approach that focuses on the child's family relationships. Third, although often filled with much wisdom and solid clinical practice, most books on treatment do not provide a detailed look at the relational complexities that follow from the trauma of incest.

The Growing Problem of Child Sexual Abuse

The social and health problem of child sexual abuse is getting worse, not better. This increase in the rates of abuse has occurred despite the dramatic increase over the past 30 years in public awareness about abuse and its effects, and in spite of the proliferation of early detection and prevention programs. Depending on the methods used to ascertain incidence and on the definitions of abuse, the most recent national estimates range from 114,000 (National Center on Child Abuse Prevention Research of the National Committee to Prevent Child Abuse [NCPCA]; Wiese & Daro, 1995) to 300,000 (National Incidence Studies [NIS-3]; Sedlak & Broadhurst, 1996) sexually abused children per year.[2] Compared to rates from 1986, this represents an increased incidence rate of up to 125% (Sedlak & Broadhurst, 1996), which parallels (actually, exceeds) the increase in all forms of maltreatment, estimated to have risen 98% since 1986 (Sedlak & Broadhurst, 1996). Prevalence statistics—determined through surveys of adults about their experiences in childhood—indicate that somewhere between 15% and 38% of adult women and about 10% of adult men report experiences of "various types of sexual victimization during childhood and adolescence" (National Clearinghouse on Child Abuse and Neglect Information, 1996, p. 1; see also important studies by Russell, 1983, 1984, and Finkelhor, Hotaling, Lewis, & Smith, 1990).

It is believed that the large majority of abused children are abused by family members (intrafamilial child sexual abuse) as opposed to persons outside the family (extrafamilial child sexual abuse). In one study (U.S. Department of Health and Human Services, National Center on Child Abuse and Neglect [NCCAN], 1996), parents made up 80% of the persons who perpetrated all types of abuse, with an additional 10% made up of

---

[2]See Appendix B to obtain information on epidemiological studies from these agencies.

other relatives.[3] In the one national study that gathered statistics on the relationship between the persons who offended and those whom they abused,[4] slightly more than one-fourth of children were sexually abused by a biological parent (Sedlak & Broadhurst, 1996). Although the data do not presently define the relationship between offending persons and abused children more specifically, a fair percentage of nonparental persons who offend are likely to be siblings, as 22% of children were abused by a person under 26 years of age. Likewise, prevalence data indicate that up to one-third of offending persons are parent figures, and all relatives combined constitute one-half of offending persons (Berliner & Elliott, 1996).

Although the finding of increased rates of abuse may be due in part to increased sensitivity and reporting of maltreatment on the part of professionals and some caretakers, the nature of the statistics "appears to herald a true rise in the scope and severity of child abuse and neglect in the United States" (Sedlak & Broadhurst, 1996, p. 17). In addition, underreporting of sexual abuse to state CPS registries—especially for middle- to upper-class families—results in estimates believed to underrepresent markedly the actual incidence of abuse (Berliner & Elliott, 1996; Peters, Wyatt, & Finkelhor, 1986), possibly by as much as two-thirds (see discussion by Sedlak & Broadhurst, 1996). In addition, a number of retrospective prevalence studies with adults who were sexually abused as children suggest that somewhere between 33% and 75% never told anyone about the abuse prior to participation in these surveys (Finkelhor, 1979; Russell, 1983, 1984), with men disclosing even less than women (Finkelhor et al., 1990). It is likely that a fair percentage of sexual abuse remains known only to the abused person and the person who offended, and may even not have been recognized as abuse by the victimized child at the time (Finkelhor & Hotaling, 1984).

Interestingly, given the current debate about the possibility of false

---

[3]However, estimates based on state reports are believed to overrepresent the frequency of intrafamilial child sexual abuse as compared to extrafamilial abuse, because extrafamilial abuse is reported to the police rather than to CPS, and there is currently "no national reporting system for crimes against children" (Berliner & Elliott, 1996, p. 51).

[4]Rather than the terms "offender" or "perpetrator," we prefer the terms "person who offended" or "family member who offended" to emphasize that the persons are not synonymous with their offending behavior. Such a distinction does not minimize the seriousness of the offending acts; rather, we believe that separating persons from their abusive acts encourages a sense of hope that they can take responsibility for ensuring that they do not offend again. Likewise, we generally use the term "abused child" rather than "victim" to denote a child who has many other characteristics and life experiences aside from having been abused and victimized.

memories of sexual abuse (Loftus & Ketcham, 1994; Yapko, 1994), one possible critique of retrospective studies might be that adult interviewees overestimate the frequency of childhood abuse. However, at least one recent *prospective* (follow-up) study of sexually abused and assaulted girls suggests that adults may retrospectively *underestimate* the frequency of abuse events. In this study, over one-third of the women did not recall childhood abuse incidents for which they had been examined at a hospital an average of 17 years earlier (Williams, 1994).

Thus, epidemiological data indicate that sexual abuse continues to occur at alarmingly high rates in the United States. Furthermore, a recent review of international abuse statistics indicated that the frequency rates of sexual abuse were not widely discrepant across 21 countries (Finkelhor, 1994). And because of the wide range of negative psychological, behavioral, and social effects of abuse on children (Berliner & Elliott, 1996), and on adults abused as children (Davies & Frawley, 1994), clinicians are likely to encounter clients who have been abused. We wrote this book with those clinicians and clients in mind.

Research Supporting a Relational Approach

Appendix A presents a summary of research that supports the relational approach to treatment of incest. However, a few central points are worth noting from the outset. First, findings on children's disclosure and recantation of abuse suggest that most children fear the relational consequences of disclosure. Elliott and Briere (1994) reported data indicating that 75% of children did not disclose the abuse within a year of the first incident, and 18% waited longer than 5 years to disclose. Berliner and Elliott (1996) note that "in 45% to 75% of all cases that come to the attention of authorities, the precipitating event is something other than the child's disclosure of abuse. Abuse may be uncovered because of suspicious behaviors or statements, medical findings of injury or infection, or because a witness interrupted the abuse, pornographic pictures were found, or an offender confessed" (p. 54). Children are reluctant to disclose because of fear of retaliation by the offending person, fear of punishment and anger on the part of nonoffending parents, and fear of precipitating negative consequences for themselves and their family members, and for the offending person (Berliner & Elliott, 1996).

Even if they do disclose, these fears may lead children to recant partially or fully. In one study of 116 confirmed cases of sexual abuse, close to

75% of children did not disclose the abuse when first questioned (Sorenson & Snow, 1991), and only 11% made unqualified disclosures. Other studies have found that between "8% and 22% of children recant true allegations of sexual abuse" (Berliner & Elliott, 1996, p. 54). Presence or absence of maternal support appears to be particularly influential in whether children initially report abuse, and whether they recant (Elliott & Briere, 1994; Lawson & Chaffin, 1992).

Children's reluctance to disclose, and their tendency to recant, contributes to an underestimation of the incidence and prevalence of sexual abuse, and, more importantly, compromises their likelihood of receiving protection and treatment at all. But more importantly from the current perspective, these data powerfully indicate that many children are so afraid of the relational impact of telling a nonoffending parent about the abuse that they are willing to suffer in silence. Clearly, therapy must address children's relational fears, whether real or unfounded, and must directly strengthen safe family relationships so that children can get the support they need from the important persons in their lives in order to heal.

Second, a number of reviews on the effects of sexual abuse have concluded that a fair percentage of sexually abused children do not exhibit clinically significant symptoms (cf. Kendall-Tackett, Williams, & Finkelhor, 1993).[5] However, few studies have rigorously assessed the signs and symptoms of *relational trauma*. We would describe some of these signs and symptoms as change in the child's sense of safety, security, and trust with family members (both offending and nonoffending); change in the child's felt ability to communicate openly with family members, and in initiation of, or response to, communication with others; and change in the child's sense of self in relation to others—that is, no longer feeling valuable, loved, cared about, and treasured. The relational approach described in this book refocuses the assessment and treatment lens from the traditional diagnostic categories of the American Psychiatric Association's *Diagnostic and Statistical Manual of Mental Disorders* (DSM) onto the nature and experience of the child's relationships.

---

[5]For an excellent review of the range of symptoms experienced by sexually abused children, see Berliner and Elliott (1996). For a wide-ranging discussion of the impact of traumatic stress, see van der Kolk, McFarlane, and Weisaeth (1996).

The Need to Address Clinical Complexity

A useful book on the treatment of families in which there has been sexual abuse must center upon how to approach the challenging relational contradictions and binds experienced by families, as well as the complicated choice points experienced by therapists who work with them. In our reading of the existing literature on treatment of sexual abuse, little space is devoted to identifying and exploring these complicated issues. Rather, books are more often written in a structured, directive, "how to" fashion meant to guide the therapist so that she or he is faced with few dilemmas and need not make as many challenging decisions with the family. Although we hope this book will assist therapists to navigate more easily the tricky waters of incest treatment, we believe the best way to assist clinicians to prepare for these waters is to provide a detailed set of maps of the range of possible "reefs," "currents," and "whirlpools" they and the families they work with may encounter, with some guidelines about how to chart their course. We base this assumption on years of teaching experience, and from training hundreds of clinicians in work with incest, in which the core questions of our trainees, from beginner to advanced, are always, "But why did you do this instead of something else?" and "But how would the approach work with *this* particular situation or *this* particular family?"

We emphasize the need for a *set* of maps, not just one, because there is no single "incest story." Although different children and families often share certain experiences, each child and his or her family's experience will also be unique. As much as possible, without becoming overly detailed or cumbersome, we have written this book in the style of themes and variations. Even with this approach, we are aware that we have not captured every possible scenario. We hope at least that in bringing the various relational issues into full view, we will assist therapists to anticipate most of the important questions.

ORGANIZATION OF THE BOOK

Part I elaborates, through a variety of approaches, the dilemmas of incest and our overall approach to them. Chapter 1 picks up where we leave off here in the Preface with an overview of the relational approach. Chapter 2 further introduces families' and therapists' dilemmas through a detailed case and commentary. Chapter 3 describes how the integration of social constructionist, feminist, and systems thinking and practice creates a flexible, comprehensive, and morally sound approach to the challenges of incest.

Part II describes the details of conducting treatment from the relational approach. Chapter 4 addresses the inherent relational complexity of the incest "story," and focuses on how to assist families to recover and expand their "stories of pride"—positive aspects of family identity, interaction, and resilience that are often submerged by the "story of shame" that is incest. In this chapter, we focus particularly on the critical role of honoring the complex web of attachments and loyalties felt by abused children and their nonoffending family members toward each other and the offending family member, and on how recognizing these seemingly contradictory feelings toward self and others eventually paves the way for moving on from (but not forgetting) the incest story.

Chapter 5 focuses on how to organize and conduct the treatment in a manner that engages the family and promotes the child's comfort and safety. Involving the child and family members as collaborators in designing their own treatment is enormously empowering to them and provides an experience that restores a sense of control and self-respect. Included here is a description of how to use multiple treatment modalities (individual, family, and group) in a manner that markedly increases the quality of information about each individual family member and the relationships among them.

Chapter 6 extends and deepens the themes introduced earlier as we discuss the details of strengthening the mother–child relationship. Here, we examine the factors that may come between parent and child—the mother's definition of herself as "cold" or unaffectionate, her difficult relationship with her own mother, her own history of abuse, gender beliefs that favor boys and men over girls and women, and various forms of denial that usually hinge on her divided loyalties between the child and the offending family member.

Chapter 7 addresses treatment of the offending family member. It describes bringing to bear the two complementary moral perspectives of justice and care, exploring and expanding the offending member's sense of self, working with him to develop empathy and a sense of others as subjects rather than objects, and including him in developing plans to safeguard the victimized child. It also includes guidelines regarding when, how, and why to conduct sessions that bring together the child and the offending family member, and for conducting an apology session.

Chapter 8 provides three case histories that further illustrate all of these issues and practices in sequence. Appendix A extends the argument for a relational approach, this time through a brief review of research on aspects of family relationships believed to enhance the abused child's resilience. We also distinguish our family-centered approach from those based on the notion of a dysfunctional "incest family." Finally, Appendix B provides a list of resources for professionals working with incest.

A note on the case material. All potentially identifying characteristics of family members have been modified to protect their privacy. We have also chosen to describe ourselves and our colleagues as "the therapist" except in the longer case examples, where the therapist is named.

Contents

PART I

Basics of the Relational Approach

Chapter One

The Relational Approach

I n this chapter, we describe the essential ideas and practices of the relational approach to the treatment of incest. We begin by identifying the central aspect of the experience of intrafamilial child sexual abuse that the relational treatment approach is designed to address, namely, the trauma caused to family relationships by the abuse and the events surrounding disclosure. This *relational trauma* has specific impacts on all family members. We then describe the range of treatment dilemmas faced by therapists as they confront the complexity of the family's experience and situation that results from this trauma. From there, we present the essential elements of the relational approach, described in detail in the remainder of the book. Finally, we end with a brief discussion of how the relational approach to treatment is supported by emerging research, and how it suggests new directions for the empirical study of sexual abuse.

INCEST AS RELATIONAL TRAUMA: THE VIEW FROM CLINICAL WORK

When a child is sexually abused, she[1] struggles with a number of relational binds, contradictions, confusions, and dilemmas. Some of these are about what to do: for instance, whether to attempt to resist the person who offended, or when this is impossible because of his threats, how to participate physically without participating emotionally. If he tells her that disclosing the abuse will break apart the family and hurt her mother and other family members, she may struggle between the desperate need to protect herself and her wish not to threaten the unity of the family. If she does decide to disclose, she may wonder if it is best to tell the nonoffending parent—who the child may fear will blame and be angry with her, or will side with the person who offended, or just not believe her—or to tell someone else and risk having the parent be angry that she wasn't told directly.

Other confusions revolve around identity and meaning: how to reconcile her experience of the offending family member as a person who in some ways seems to love her, and even takes care of her, with her experience of him as someone who violates her trust, her personhood, her body; how to view the nonoffending parent as someone who can protect her in the future, when she hasn't in the past; how to view herself as a girl her own age, after participating in activities she may know are meant for adults; how to feel about her body once she has been violated; how to think that she is worth loving and protecting, and is a good person, when she has been abused; how to think of her whole family—as a good, safe family, or a bad, dangerous family.

The nonoffending parent—usually a mother or someone in the mothering role—faces numerous conflicting emotional and relational demands once she knows about the abuse. Her primary challenge centers on how best to protect her abused child as well as the other children. She may struggle about whether to report the abuse, especially if her partner has been intimidating or violent in the past, or, once the abuse has come to light, has threatened harm if it is disclosed to authorities. If she has had negative experiences with the police or child welfare, or knows other families that have, she may believe more damage will be incurred to the child and family by reporting than if she tries to handle the situation herself. She may have heard about families being torn apart after disclosure, children placed in foster care, and nonoffending parents being prosecuted for neglect. She may worry about the financial and material effects her family will suffer once the person who offended is removed from the home or goes

---

[1](footnote from page 3) We use the pronoun "she" to refer to the abused child because the most recent incidence and prevalence statistics indicate the majority of incestuously abused children are female (Finkelhor et al., 1990; Sedlack & Broadhurst, 1996), and to avoid the awkwardness of using both the male and female pronouns repeatedly throughout the text. However, these dilemmas are also faced by male abused children.

to jail. If she does report and the person who offended is removed from the home, she may wonder whether or what to tell the nonabused children. Although she may wish to reach out for help from others, she may also be anxious about the blame and social stigma that she, her daughter, and whole family will incur if the abuse becomes known to extended family members, neighbors, the school, and the community.

The nonoffending mother may also struggle with mixed feelings and competing loyalties toward the child and the person who offended. She may wonder whom to believe. And, like her daughter, she may struggle with issues of meaning and identity: how to feel about this man (or boy, if the person who offended is her son or nephew) who has hurt her daughter and betrayed them all; how to view her daughter—whether to blame her even in some small way, or to see her truly as a victim and a survivor; how to see herself as a parent—and whether to blame herself for the abuse, given that she was not able to prevent it up until now; how to view her marriage if the person who offended was her partner—as a relationship based on love or on a lie; and how to view the family as a whole—as one with many good qualities and times alongside this terrible chapter, or as fundamentally flawed.

Once the abuse comes to light, the adult who offended also may experience contradictory feelings and agendas. His dominant experience may be a mixture of fear, rationalizing and justifying his behavior, and a sense of shame. He may struggle with whether to acknowledge what he did despite the legal consequences or to ignore again the well-being of the child and deny the allegations. Both adult and juvenile persons who offend may recognize that they need treatment, yet may be afraid to engage in it for a variety of possible reasons, including fear that information revealed in the course of therapy will compromise their legal cases or further affect how family members view them. If the person who offended was abused as a child, he may be anxious about facing and discussing his own history of abuse; and often, whether he himself was abused or not, the person who offended may fear coming to terms with, and talking about, his sexuality.

Treatment Challenges

Therapists struggle with a wide range of choice points that can make working with sexually abused children and their families extremely confusing and challenging. For instance, clinicians need to balance a collaborative approach—empowering families to make decisions for themselves, respecting their expertise about themselves and their suggestions about how to solve problems, identifying and building on families' existing strengths and resources—with ensuring that the abused children and other nonoffending family members will be safe from further abuse. In other words, how does the therapist handle moments when the family's proposed solutions greatly conflict with "expert knowledge" and experience? Another challenge centers on creating a space for the abused children and other nonoffending family members to talk about their enduring loyalties and attachment to the persons who offended, while at the same time helping them reshape the nature and physical proximity of their relationships with the persons who offended so that safety can be guaranteed. How can therapists help families redefine themselves once there has been such an enormous breach of trust? How do we create a morally sound therapy—where blame for the abuse is accurately placed on the shoulders of the person who offended—while at the same time allowing nonoffending family members to voice and struggle with their shame and self-blame, and give them the opportunity to recognize what they could do differently in the future so as to prevent further abuse?

On a more pragmatic level, other choice points include how to balance attention to the abuse with the often multiple other needs of the child and other family members; how to handle the sometimes severe individual symptoms of the traumatized child within a family therapy framework; conversely, whether or how to proceed if the child has no signs or symptoms of distress; what to do if it's still not clear that the abuse occurred; how to organize the treatment—whom to see first and next; what to talk about with all the nonoffending family members present, with just the parent and abused child, with the child alone; whether to work with the person who offended, and whether to have sessions that bring the person who offended together with the abused child; what to do with important information a child provides in an individual session—whether or how to tell the parent who must protect her; how to balance the child's right to privacy with the need to strengthen her connection to the nonoffending parent.

Therapists also face a number of potential impasses created by the complex relationships between themselves, the family, and the "larger system" of professionals involved in cases of sexual abuse. These include balancing issues of social control—for instance, your role as a legally mandated reporter of abuse and as the writer of case notes that could be subpoenaed in a trial—with your role as a trusted therapist. How can you keep clear about your role as a therapist with the family when the social service and legal professionals involved with a case may hope the therapy can double as a forensic investigation? How can you maintain clarity in the middle of fractured families and polarized positions, both within the family and, often, among the social agencies that form the system surrounding the family?

And therapists also have to manage the strong emotions and other reactions evoked in them in the course of working with sexual abuse. How do you recognize but contain personal responses when you hear about extremely upsetting events, or when parents describe beliefs that go against your values? For instance, how should you respond when a woman firmly voices beliefs about child rearing, or about the degree of protection or power to which men versus women are entitled—beliefs that differ drastically from your own, and that seem to put her and the child at risk?

WHAT IS THE RELATIONAL APPROACH?

In a sentence, the relational approach to treatment is designed to strengthen the safe, protective relationships between the child and her family members and to reempower these individuals and relationships so that the family can be a safe, nurturing place. Table 1.1 lists the central goals of this approach. The perspectives and practices summarized here will assist you in negotiating the challenging dilemmas and promoting the goals of treatment by honoring the inherently complex nature of the experience of incest. The remainder of the book, particularly Part II, takes up each idea and practice and illustrates them with many clinical vignettes.

Given some variation, clinicians working with children and families in which there has been sexual abuse share beliefs about the goals and treatment practices for the abused child, as well as for the offending family member (cf. Bentovim, 1998; Bentovim, Elton, Hildebrand, & Vizard, 1988; Cohen & Mannarino, 1993; Friedrich, 1990, 1995; Gelinas, 1988; Gil, 1996; Gil & Johnson, 1993; Jenkins, 1990; Mandell et al., 1989; Miller & Dwyer, 1997; Sgroi, 1982; Trepper & Barrett, 1989).[2] However, there are important distinctions that center around (1) which aspects of therapeutic intervention are emphasized, (2) how different treatment modalities are utilized and connected to each other, (3) the degree to which the therapy is structured, and (4) different ideas about what constitutes family therapy.

---

[2]The focus of this book is not to compare the relational approach point by point to other models of child sexual abuse treatment. However, we wish to acknowledge the important work of these authors.

TABLE 1.1. Treatment Goals of the Relational Approach to Incest

The abused child

- To develop *personal agency*—the ability to affect what happens to her in relationships and to control outcomes in her life
- To not blame herself for the abuse
- To reconnect with a trustworthy family member (usually her mother)
- To become asymptomatic in terms of emotional and behavioral sequelae

The nonoffending parent

- To be a trustworthy parent, who makes morally sound and protective decisions on behalf of her child
- To be able to tolerate expression of a range of feelings from the child
- To identify, clarify, and accept her many feelings about the offending person

The person who offended

- To take responsibility for the abuse
- To show empathy for the child
- To participate in generating a safety plan

The family as a whole

- To regain and build upon stories of pride without diminishing the significance of the incest "story"
- To resume and/or strengthen relationships with supportive others in the extended family and community
- To become a place of safety, nurturance, and growth—protection from the possibility of future abuses

These distinctions are clarified in the description of the particular theoretical underpinnings and practices of the relational approach.

Family as the Central Focus for Treatment: Strengthening the Child's Safe and Protective Relationships

The essence or major focus of the relational approach to intrafamilial child sexual abuse is to restore and strengthen the child's relationships with protective family members—especially the mother in most cases—and to clarify and make safe the child's relationship with the person who offended. Strengthening the mother–daughter relationship and other of the child's safe relationships is essential to her recovery when difficulties in the mother–daughter bond predate the abuse, when difficulties arise as a result of the abuse, as well as when their relationship is fairly strong but challenged by the issues and events surrounding disclosure.

One illustrative example involved a first-generation immigrant family from the Dominican Republic that included a 12-year-old daughter, mother, and stepfather. The mother and daughter in this family had a problematic attachment that preceded the daughter's abuse by the stepfather. The mother spoke directly about how, from early on in the child's life, she had always found it difficult to be affectionate with her. This sense of being "cold" (her word) with her daughter stood in stark contrast to her clearly demonstrated love and affection for her husband.

Although the work of building a stronger mother–daughter bond had many facets, one important piece was identifying the disappointment and sadness the mother experienced about how her own mother had mothered her. Once treatment established the connection between how she was mothered and its effects on her mothering, the meaning of her mothering changed. She now approached her attempts to mother her daughter the way she wished she had been mothered as a means both to provide more care for her daughter and to soothe and make up for her own disappointments in how she was raised. Ultimately, their bond increased sufficiently so that the mother could support her daughter through the trial of the husband/stepfather, in which the daughter was required to testify.

Family Treatment and Individual Symptoms

The emphasis on strengthening safe, supportive relationships is in contrast to a therapy that focuses primarily on individual treatment of the child to eliminate her psychological and behavioral symptoms; that is, a core assumption is that unless the therapist works with the family to enhance the child's protective relationships, it may be more difficult for the child to recover from her individual symptoms and to sustain this improvement. The relational approach is as concerned with reducing or eliminating the child's individual symptoms as are approaches that highlight individual therapy for the child, but it holds that such improvement occurs primarily as the result of interventions targeted to clarify and/or improve (as appropriate) family relationships. In this way, we place the "interpersonal aspects of the trauma" of intrafamilial sexual abuse front and center (van der Kolk, McFarlane, & van der Hart, 1996, p. 420).

When a child describes or displays symptoms, or when they are reported by the nonoffending parent, we work with the child in both individual and family sessions to understand the nature and extent of these symptoms, as well as when and where they occur (e.g., the pattern), and to identify what the child and family may already be doing to lessen or stop them, at least temporarily. These existing strengths are then built upon in an individualized plan to monitor and interrupt the symptoms. The key to our approach to ameliorating the child's psychological symptoms is that we work with the child and family to *use the symptoms as signals* for the child to connect with a supportive adult (and sometimes also a responsible older sibling) for support, comfort, and soothing. We have found that with this approach, the child's symptoms resolve without recourse to specialized cognitive-behavioral or other therapeutic techniques (Deblinger & Heflin, 1996).

One family we saw included 6-year-old twin girls, their father, and his wife of approximately 1 year. One girl, who had been abused by the boyfriend of the biological mother, was now acting out sexually with her sister. The stepmother, in an attempt to be a protective mother figure, responded punitively to the acting-out stepdaughter. We first helped her and the father view the daughter's sexualized behavior as driven by anxiety and a need for connection that derived from her abrupt and confusing separation from her biological mother and grandmother. Next, we assisted the child to identify the early physiological signs of anxiety that preceded her sexual acting out, and suggested that at those moments she go to her parents for a hug. The general plan was first suggested in an individual session with the acting-out child, and the details were refined in a family session, with everyone contributing ideas.

Family Treatment and Sense of Self

Family treatment is essential for the child to move on from the abuse experience with minimal negative impact to her sense of self. The child's sense of self—including her self-concept, self-worth, self-awareness, sense of continuity, sense of agency and control, and sense of coherence (Harter, 1998)—is greatly affected by how family members view and interact with her (Harter, 1987, 1990, 1999). In families in which there has been incest, parents and siblings sometimes take a blaming attitude toward the abused child. The abused child comes to see herself in terms of family members' attitudes, which are reinforced in daily interactions (Cole & Putnam, 1992; Harter, 1998, 1999). Thus, although individual and group therapy can assist the child to understand how her negative sense of self derives in part from others' negative descriptions, and can assist her to develop more positive self-accounts, continued exposure to the family's negative perspectives can neutralize gains made in these other therapeutic modalities. By assisting family members to articulate more positive descriptions of the abused child both in and out of therapy sessions, and by strengthening the relationships between the child and family members, these relationships can serve as an ongoing source of positive interpersonal experiences. The child's emerging, positive self-account is thereafter validated and strengthened by her daily, significant social context, and not just in the far less frequent, and less naturalistic, context of therapy.

In one family, the mother was able to stop holding her daughter responsible for the abuse inflicted by the stepfather only after a thorough exploration of the ways the mother assumed she was responsible for the abuse she herself suffered at the hands of her own uncle. Locating her self-blaming premise in the larger frame of how women often take responsibility for the abusive actions of men connected her to the larger community of women and decreased her immobilizing shame. In turn, this allowed her to stop blaming her daughter, and to notice and support her positive qualities.

Family Treatment and Long-Term Adjustment

Assisting the entire family to overcome the effects of abuse better ensures that the child's most important social context is prepared to help her sustain recovery during the course of therapy and long after it ends. Because the abuse will have different meanings for the child throughout her development, it is important that she have an adult she can turn to whenever she needs help with her feelings. For instance, the child's memories of the abuse may remain fairly dormant until she reaches puberty or enters a sexual relationship. At this time, she may become flooded with images and feelings related to the abuse. The relational approach to treatment includes explicit work around preparing the nonoffending mother to respond supportively to the new or repeated concerns the child may experience as she matures.

Family Treatment and Other Members' Recovery

Family-centered treatment also benefits other family members, who may also be traumatized or otherwise affected, and in a manner that is well coordinated and consistent with the treatment of the child.

Gary was the 4-year-old brother of an abused girl with whom we were working. The father had abused the daughter 2 years earlier, and until treatment began, Gary seemed to have adequately adjusted to the father's absence. His adjustment was aided by the family's openly talking about missing the father and by continued contact with the paternal grandparents. However, in the last few weeks, Gary had begun talking more about missing him and was acting aggressively at home and in school.

In a session with his mother, he spoke of how his siblings hit him a lot. And in a session alone, he drew a picture of monsters that were beating, hitting, and generally frightening him. When the therapist asked if there was anyone who could stop the monsters, he said, "My daddy." When asked if there was anyone else, he said, "the police." The therapist then asked if his mommy could stop them. He said no. The therapist asked, "Do you think someone could teach Mommy how to stop them?" He asked, "Who?" and the therapist suggested she might be able to help. After the little boy suggested that his mother might get a gun and shoot the monsters, the therapist said, "Well, I think she might stop them if she says, 'No one is allowed to hit my son Gary!' "

Together, Gary and the therapist restated this sentence with conviction and emotion several times. Gary then agreed for the therapist to share this with his mother. The therapist and child brought the mother into the session, showed her the picture of the monsters, and shared with her the idea of how she could protect Gary from them. The mother thought it was a good idea and practiced under Gary's guidance just how to say it.

Gary's mother and the therapist spoke further about how to stop the hitting among the siblings. In subsequent sessions, she reported that Gary's behavior in school and at home had dramatically improved, and that there was much less hitting among the children.

All nonoffending family members are affected to some extent by the incest, and relationships among them are often characterized by anger, bitterness, sadness, disconnection, and loss of trust. Often, members have not openly discussed with each other their feelings about incest-related events, fearing a negative response. Family therapy assists nonoffending family members to understand each others' experiences, to clear up misunderstandings among members, and to jointly mourn this chapter in the shared story of their lives, so that they can begin to rebuild connection and trust. In some cases, these conversations will also include the offending family member, as we describe later.

Family Treatment and Long-Term Safety

In addition to its effectiveness in addressing efficiently both relational and individual trauma, the relational approach is critical for families in which the person who offended or others who could perpetrate abuse still have access to the child. Aside from removing the child from the home, which may create more trauma than the abuse itself, work with the nonoffending parent is critical to protecting the child from future abuse. A core focus of the relational approach is to assist the child and nonoffending family members to cope with the conflicts and contradictions surrounding how they feel about the person who offended; not revealing these feelings can set the stage for allowing the offending member back into the family in unsafe ways. How to understand that they still love and feel attached to him despite what he did, how to square their fear and rage with memories of times when he was protective, rather than someone whom they needed protection *from*, become critical issues to approach in intrafamilial sexual abuse treatment.

Whether the person who offended returns to the home after treatment (more likely in the case of juvenile offending persons than adults), is involved with the family but is physically separated from them, or is never seen by the child again, therapy needs to help the child and others sort out their complex feelings toward him, and, if he lives near the child, to develop a clear plan to prevent further abuse. When possible and appropriate, the relational approach also includes intensive therapy with the person who offended, and if this results in his taking complete responsibility for the abuse and developing true empathy for the child he abused and the others he hurt, treatment may include family sessions that allow him to apologize directly to the child.

The Critical Role of a Collaborative Stance

If treatment is to be successful, it must be construed as a journey of the therapist and family together. The nature of the abuse experience especially requires a more collaborative approach to treatment. One of the core experiences of abused children and their nonoffending family members is that the person who offended exercised absolute power over them by acting on his desires in a manner that negatively affected their lives and integrity. Often, one way he accomplishes this is to cut off the child from sources of protection and support. Therefore, an effective therapy must reempower and reconnect the child and other nonoffending family members so that they can directly affect the conditions in their lives.

To achieve this outcome, therapy for incest requires a high degree of respectful collaboration and connection between the therapist and family. Much of this collaboration centers on decisions regarding the process and organization of each session, and of the therapy as a whole. That is, the relational therapist attends not only to the content of what family members say, or to the particular issues and questions raised by either family member or therapist, but also thinks about how to engage family members in decisions about whom to involve in therapy first and next, which topics to discuss within each session, when to stop talking about the abuse and when to revisit it, how to work with other professionals, and which therapeutic modality to use when. This attention to the collaborative organization of therapy results in the entire encounter between clients and therapist being respectful, relational, and moral.

For example, we may discuss with the family whether or not to invite to a meeting the involved child welfare workers and lawyers in order to clarify legal issues and treatment expectations. In many cases, we discuss with the family whether there are extended family members who could be helpful, and whether and how they should be invited into the therapy. In one situation, a stepfather abused a child and her biological father did not provide emotional support, something the child desperately craved. After discussing with the family who might most effectively engage this father, the child's mother contacted her ex-husband's mother and sister and invited them to a family session. The father heard about this meeting, learned what was going on in the therapy, came to better appreciate the trauma his daughter had experienced, and as a result became much more responsive to his daughter's needs.

Just as collaboration is critical with other family members, we engage the person who offended collaboratively as well. For instance, although we design the apology session (or an apology letter) between the person who offended and the child largely based on what the abused child says she needs to hear, we also discuss with the person who offended what he believes would be important to say to her, so that it becomes completely clear that she did not cause the abuse and that he is truly sorry for the pain he caused her. When treating an offending person, we also coauthor with him letters to supervising agencies regarding his progress in treatment, and, as we do in sessions with other family members, we invite the person who offended to tell us how he feels the therapy is going in general, to codirect the flow and content of any particular session, and to participate in decisions with us about what information would best be transferred from an individual session to a session with other family members.

Creating this collaborative approach—and from the family's point of view, embracing this approach—can be especially challenging in work with incest. Families may have been mandated or at least directed, to therapy, sometimes as a condition of being reunited after children have been removed by CPS, and so initially may feel they have to "cooperate" with the therapist—a stance quite different from the active participation and joint decision making implied by collaboration. Families, concerned that they will experience yet another betrayal, may have initial difficulty trusting the therapist not only because of the betrayal experienced at the hands of the person who offended, but also if the responses of CPS, the police, and other professionals following disclosure of the abuse were unwittingly not sensitive and respectful. Family members, who may also feel at an all-time low in terms of their sense of pride and trust in their own judgment, as well as disconnected from each other and their usual sources of support in extended family and community, may look to the therapist to make decisions for them. The therapist may also be concerned at times about the quality of judgment and degree of resourcefulness of the adult family members, especially regarding future protection of the child. However, these challenges to creating collaboration and reempowering families are precisely one of the key foci of the relational approach to therapy. In short, the dilemma that must be approached is how to sustain an empowering collaborative stance toward the family in the face of an egregious violation of the child's safety.

Use of Multiple Modalities

In the relational approach, therapists see family members both in individual and conjoint family sessions, and hold groups for children and nonoffending parents when possible. One therapist either does the work in all the modalities, or, if there is more than one therapist, each observes the work of the other. This ensures that all the information is held in one individual or collective "mind."

Why use multiple therapeutic modalities? Various therapeutic/relational contexts allow different information to emerge. Often, especially at the beginning of therapy, the relationship between the child and the nonoffending parent may be quite strained. The nonoffending parent may be extremely worried about the child, feel guilty about the abuse, and also feel angry at the child. As a result, the child may feel constrained from freely talking in the presence of the parent. Individual sessions with the child, away from troubled interactions with parents, may allow a less pressured setting in which to reflect upon the child's wishes, feelings, and concerns. However, once she finds and defines her voice, the therapist turns the child back to the family and works with her to express herself directly or with the therapist's assistance. Although the therapist needs to attend to and work with the ways in which the child repeats in the therapeutic relationship patterns in which she engages with her parents, the relational approach focuses not on interpreting transference but on preparing the child to go back to the family and take an active role in changing the quality of these family relationships.

Likewise, the parent may have information or feelings that would be more appropriately discussed without the child present. However, the relational therapist always looks for ways to build on the information provided by the parent in these individual sessions to enhance her relationship with her child. Thus, this approach does not involve ongoing, separate individual therapies with family members. Instead, individual sessions of varying length are used as part of the family therapy. Ultimately, the goal of individual sessions is the same as the family sessions—to clarify and strengthen family relationships, largely through opening communication between family members.

Transfer of Information among Modalities

The relational approach is recursive in that information is transferred from one therapy modality to another and back again. The transfer of information from one modality to another is accomplished through a practice called the "Decision Dialogue," in which the family member and therapist discuss what information is to be brought back into another modality. When a family member does not want information to be shared with others—for instance, when a child is reluctant to share information from an individual session with her parent in a family session—the therapist focuses on the family member's reluctance to speak. It is through these Decision Dialogues that relational dilemmas and impasses are often most clearly revealed.

The Decision Dialogue also promotes personal agency in the child by including her in all decisions about what to share and not share with other family members. For an abused child whose agency was subjugated to the will of an adult, the invitation to decide whether or how to share highly charged information may be her first opportunity to begin regaining a sense of personal control over her relationship with others. Although the therapist's opinions may differ from the child's about what might be best to tell other family members, these opinions are discussed but not imposed upon her. Aside from information that must be transferred because not to do so would endanger the child, the child has the final say about what will be transferred from individual to family sessions.

Thus, the Decision Dialogue is one of the key practices of the approach and serves multiple purposes. As the vehicle for linking the modalities, it encourages personal agency in formerly disempowered family members and helps sustain a client-determined agenda.

Inviting Complex Relational Descriptions

As noted at the beginning of this chapter, many of the confusions and relational binds experienced by abused children center on how they feel about the persons who offended, themselves, and the nonoffending family members. To help the child prevent self-blame and help her to relieve often intense emotional confusion, the therapist assists her to bring forth her complex and often contradictory feelings. For instance, typically, the abused child feels (and is told by the nonoffending parent or the professionals she encounters) that it is "OK" or "normal" to have negative feelings about the person who offended, but she is troubled by her continuing positive feelings of love, fondness, and concern about his well-being. Furthermore, because a child may receive support from others in her role as victim, she may be afraid to reveal that she holds positive feelings toward the person who abused her. She may even have enjoyed aspects of her relationship with the person who offended, including some of the sexual activity, and so may worry that this means she is responsible for having been abused. By normalizing a wide range of possible feelings towards the person who offended, as well as physical sensations she had during the abuse, the therapist helps the child to make sense of her total experience. Therefore, although the therapist explores and encourages the expression of pain, hurt, and betrayal that abused children usually express, he or she must also remain alert to the presence of other feelings that the child may not feel as comfortable about sharing.

For example, after a child described in graphic detail the emotional and psychological injury her uncle caused her, we inquired whether she ever felt other, positive feelings. When she quickly responded with a description of how he had been her favorite uncle, we were able to comment on how it might be confusing to know him in such different ways and to have such different feelings. It is this type of observation children often experience as relieving and freeing, in that both their emotional realities are honored and neither must be chosen over the other. When the child believes that one reality of her experience must be denied in order to maintain intrapsychic coherence and her relational bonds, she is at risk of acting out or developing other symptoms.

Similarly, therapy helps the child express conflicting feelings about the nonoffending parent (or both parents, when the person who offended was a sibling or other child relative rather than a parent), particularly when the child tried to tell the parent of the abuse or the parent did not respond in a protective fashion immediately upon finding out. In contrast to her feelings about the person who offended, the child usually believes it is acceptable to feel and show love and connection toward the nonoffending parent, but not anger, resentment, distrust, or fear. One child spoke of having "slips" whenever she expressed anger toward her mother. The risk of directly expressing anger was too threatening to her, as she had already "lost" one parent (the person who abused her), and she feared her anger might alienate the other. Another child feared that her mother, who missed her son, who had been removed from the home after his abuse of the daughter was disclosed, would be angry with her if she expressed any angry feelings.

Honoring the Nonoffending Mother's Attachment to the Person Who Offended

To accomplish the treatment goals for the nonoffending parent—typically, the mother—it is critical to bring forth the bond between the mother and the offending family member. This is an essential step both to restoring the bond between mother and child, and to ensuring that the mother makes decisions that protect her child. At first glance, it might seem more effective for the therapist to focus on supporting the mother in her anger, rage, and sense of betrayal toward the person who abused her and her child, as a way of empowering her to protect the child. Although it is certainly critical to give the mother space to describe her anger and betrayal, it is more likely that the unstated and almost always shameful attachment to the abusing partner will inhibit both the mother's moral clarity and her unambiguous emotional support for her child. The degree to which the therapist brings forth a woman's attachment to the offending partner (or to the offending child, in the case of a juvenile person who offended), normalizes it, and models holding its inherent contradictions, is the extent to which a mother begins to experience clarity instead of confusion, strength instead of shame.

Although this may sound like a romanticized, unrealistic description of the therapy process—or even sound risky in that it provides validation for the woman's continued feelings of attachment to the person who offended, our repeated experience is that when we trust the process and accept these feelings, the mothers do not fail to protect and connect with their children. Of course, one key to the success of this approach is to distinguish clearly between *feelings* of attachment and *actions* that bring the person who offended unsafely in proximity to the child. Nevertheless, some therapists in our workshops often initially express concern about this approach to working with the nonoffending mother. We often are asked,

"What do you do with the mothers who knew and didn't act?" and "What do you do with the mothers who still don't support their daughters?" After 2 days of extensive videotaped examples, these participants understand what we experience time and again. Mothers who are withdrawn, withholding, overly critical, and seemingly not affectionate with their daughters respond to our acknowledgment that as women they may love, miss, and long for the man who has so betrayed both them and their children. And when these feelings are acknowledged and the woman is not condemned for having them, when her shameful secret attachment is honored, she is able to respond in her role as mother differently. For as is true of people more generally, she is better able to act from a position of strength, which in turn derives from self-acceptance and self-respect.

The debilitating effects of feelings of shame and confusion are captured by one woman who, after acknowledging how much she found herself missing her partner who had extensively abused her preadolescent daughter, asked the therapist if she was crazy. Only after describing the full range of her feeling towards this man—including powerful positive memories as well as the memories of abuse and betrayal—could this mother clearly decide the future of the relationship with a man with whom she had vowed to share a life. Only after hearing from the therapist how normal was her capacity to experience opposite feelings about the same person could she sort through her options and make a clear moral choice in behalf of protecting her children.

The experience of accepting her many complex feelings toward the person who offended also expands the nonoffending mother's tolerance for the many complex feelings her child may hold toward her, toward the person who offended, and toward herself. The extent to which a mother can tolerate and understand the child's often intense mixed feelings about her and the other people in her life often determines the extent to which the child feels safe expressing these feelings to her rather than acting them out.

Building the Offending Person's Capacity for Empathy

In our work with offending persons, we listen carefully to their narratives of the abuse for signs that their focus includes any empathic understanding of the impact of their actions upon the child—or whether the focus remains upon them, their shame, their loss, and their suffering following disclosure. For example, in one instance, a man expressed remorse immediately and said that he was not the kind of man who would do such a thing. He was terribly upset, explaining that no one would believe him capable of such an act, and that though he was drunk, fondling his stepdaughter was completely alien to how he and others saw him. His entire narrative was about him. As we explored his relationship more generally with his wife and her daughter, we learned that he often viewed each of them as an extension of his needs. Only after bringing forth his premises about the roles and privileges of each gender were both he and his wife able to have a different conversation about their relationship and his relationship with her daughter. As this man began to reflect on his beliefs about gender and power, which up until that moment he had never articulated to himself or to others, he could begin to consider how others felt as a result of his abusive behavior. He then directed the therapeutic conversation further into the details of the abuse, noting periodically with a sense of his own surprise that he had never really thought about his stepdaughter's experience of it.

In addition to bringing forth the gender and power premises that sanction seeing women and girls (or boys) as objects for sexual gratification rather than as complete persons, relational therapy slowly "unpacks" or examines the abusive acts "frame-by-frame" and raises questions that require the person who offended to focus on the experience of the abused child. The empathic imagining of the abused child's experience is essential for all persons who offended, especially for those who themselves were abused as children, as they may assume that their abuse experience was identical to that which they incurred in the child. Although the therapist is also interested in the offending person's experience of the abuse and the impact of disclosure from his point of view, and is concerned with his psychological and emotional adjustment, he or she can never lose sight of the offending person's responsibility for the abuse, which he grasps most powerfully once he can "see" the full impact of his actions on the abused child.

A subsequent important step in treatment of the person who offended, and of the entire family, is to plan an apology session. In this process the person who offended must think about what he wants to say, and what meaning his apology will hold for the abused child, and, consistent with the relational approach, also for the children who were not abused, and the nonoffending parent/partner. When the person who offended is not available for an apology session—either because he is imprisoned, has been ruled by a judge not to be allowed in physical proximity to the child, is in another state, or the child or nonoffending parent do not want him physically present for a session, the therapist communicates with him through letters. Importantly, the therapist does not allow conjoint sessions with the person who offended and the abused child until he convincingly accepts complete responsibility and demonstrates empathy for the abused child.

The offending persons also participate in creating a safety plan. This is often experienced as a healthy form of empowerment for a person who has used power as a form of domination rather than to be protective. In moving from dialogue to action, the offending person has a tangible means to express new ways of being a man. He must recognize the real threat his abusive behavior poses. It is an opportunity to focus exclusively on the needs of the child he abused.

In cases in which the nature of abuse is chronic and obsessional, and it is clear that programs of cognitive restructuring and behavioral reconditioning are indicated, the offending person is referred for these specialized treatments.

INCEST AS RELATIONAL TRAUMA: THE VIEW FROM RESEARCH

In this chapter, we have argued from clinical observations and a relational approach to treatment that intrafamilial child sexual abuse is most parsimoniously viewed fundamentally as a relational problem. Whatever the type and degree of individual symptoms experienced by the child, incest inevitably traumatizes her relationships and those of all members of the family; that is, incest is at base a betrayal of the child's and nonoffending family members' primary relationships. It affects and is affected by the child's and family's relationships to the persons involved in their lives. And it is most directly "caused" by the offending person's *relational premises*—articulated verbally, or nonverbally—through his choice[3] of abusive action: premises about power, sexuality, and the nature of his relationships with the child and other family members.

In privileging the relational context, we move away from the research literature's diagnosis-driven focus on the pathology of the victimized child. We emphasize that the psychological effects of abuse go beyond the cognitive, emotional, and behavioral disturbances highlighted in this literature. In fact, the dominant focus on individual symptomatology is contradicted by other findings that question its ubiquity. This focus on symptoms largely neglects the potentially enormous impact of abuse on how children experi-

---

[3]We view all abusive action as a choice. Although some persons who offended may experience their behavior as compulsive and out of their control, in our view, their minimum responsibility is to seek help in controlling these impulses.

ence their most significant interpersonal relationships. Although a growing literature documents incidence of individual sequelae of abuse, two rather striking major conclusions from this body of research support a treatment focus on the abused child's family relationships, rather than solely on his or her symptoms.

First, the variability of symptom clusters across children and studies suggests that "there is no evidence of a single 'child sexual abuse syndrome' " (Crittenden, 1996, p. 166); that is, from the point of view of the clinician, the most important finding to date on short-term effects is the "absence of any specific syndrome in children who have been sexually abused and no single traumatizing process" (Kendall-Tackett et al., 1993, p. 164). No one symptom has been found in all or even the majority of sexually abused children.

Furthermore, a fair percentage of abused children appear to be asymptomatic: Studies have reported rates between 21% and 49% of children with no symptoms (Kendall-Tackett et al., 1993). Berliner and Elliott (1996) write, "As a group, sexually abused children do not self-report clinically significant levels of distress on symptom checklist measures of depression, anxiety, and self-esteem, and often do not differ from comparison groups of nonabused children on these measures" (p. 55).

Although a variety of methodological explanations have been offered to explain the lower than expected rates of individual symptomatology in sexually abused children (Kendall-Tackett et al., 1993; Cole & Putnam, 1992), it may be that the critical variable in determining symptom severity and duration is *how the family responds to the abuse*. For example, whereas many clinicians find that sexually abused children engage in some degree of self-blame and experience loss of self-esteem, empirical studies have generally been equivocal regarding the negative impact of abuse on the child's sense of self (Berliner & Elliott, 1996; Hunter, Goodwin, & Wilson, 1992; Kendall-Tackett et al., 1993). Although this lack of clear findings may be methodologically based, it is also possible that variability in impact on self-worth *depends on the degree to which potentially protective family members side with or blame the child*. Whereas the impact on self-concept may not show up immediately for abused children, over time, children who are emotionally unsupported and blamed for the abuse might eventually link the abuse to their sense of self. In contrast, for those who are supported and reassured as to their blamelessness immediately or soon after the disclosure of abuse, their self-concept might develop relatively untrammeled by the abuse. In fact, for the latter group of children, the groundswell of emotional care and support might affirm their sense of self in positive ways. This view gains support from Harter's (1990, 1998, 1999) theory that the responses of the social world to the child greatly shape the development of her or his self-concept and self-worth; and from the set of findings that parental support at the time of disclosure affects recovery from abuse (Conte & Schuerman, 1987; Everson, Hunter, Runyan, Edelsohn, & Coulter, 1989).

The concept of incest as relational trauma points not only to the importance of a relational treatment but also to new directions for research. Clinical assessment and research that examines abused children's ideas and feelings about their family relationships and about relationships in general may find that a fair percentage of those deemed asymptomatic in terms of traditional diagnostic and other individually based categories suffer greatly in their relationships and in their self-experience regarding relationships. Treatment needs to address these relationships and children's representations of them. That's what this book is about.

Chapter Two

The Relational Approach in Action

In Chapter 1, we introduced some of the painful contradictions, loyalty binds, and bewildering dilemmas families face when a family member abuses a child. In this chapter, we present a detailed account of one family's experience. We include portions of dialogue from therapy sessions in an attempt to capture the raw emotional quality of their experience. We chose to present this family because its members faced so many of the typical conflicts and struggles that follow from incest, including the following:

- A mother's confusion about what to do once she discovers the abuse: how to protect her daughter and report the offending stepfather while valiantly trying not to upset the other children and her ailing parents (an honorable intention but an impossible bind that ultimately led her not to report in time, and to be charged with neglect)
- A child's conflict around whether to disclose the abuse, and to whom
- Despite her hurt and anger toward the person who offended, a child's secret feelings of continued attachment and even concern toward him

- A child's conflicts over whether to tell her mother the fear and anger she feels toward her
- A mother's complex and confusing feelings toward the person who offended

In this chapter, we also comment on the therapeutic choice points we faced in working with this family. Included in these choice points are the following:

- Whom to see first—mother or abused child?
- Issues around talking about abuse, including how to talk about the abuse without unduly upsetting or even retraumatizing the child; how much to talk about the abuse versus other issues the family faces; how best to introduce the topic of abuse or whether to talk about the abuse at all; and how to share this rationale with a child
- How to address a parent's upset with her abused child—about the disclosure, or problem behaviors—while assisting mother and daughter to strengthen their relationship
- How to use individual sessions in a manner that promotes, rather than interrupts, the goal of strengthening the child's relationship with her mother
- How to widen the relational focus of the therapeutic conversation so as to address the complex web of family loyalties
- How to balance an approach that values identifying and amplifying parents' existing strengths, knowledge, and other personal resources with the occasional need to address styles of parenting that seem unproductive and possibly even harmful to the child
- When to terminate, and how to create a plan for continued access to therapy that allows family members to feel supported as they negotiate the challenges of family life following incest disclosure

We hope the reader emerges from reading this chapter with a vivid picture of the emotional struggles of families in which incest has occurred and a sense of how therapy can address these struggles and dilemmas. We also hope that the verbatim case material and our explanations will provide a window into the "nitty gritty" of the family's experiences and the ways in which therapy theory and practices are translated into the all-important micro moves of treatment.

Judy and her children, a Polish American working-class family, were referred to us by the child advocacy center after Judy was charged with neglect of her 10-year-old daughter, Laurie. Judy was extremely nervous during our first meeting. She could barely sit still as she described the ordeal she and her children had been through since Laurie disclosed that her stepfather, Tom, had been sexually abusing her on a regular basis for the past year. Judy explained that one night she awoke and noticed that Tom was not in bed with her. She went to look for him and discovered him leaving Laurie's bedroom. Judy said that because she herself had been sexually abused as a child by her cousin, she immediately grew suspicious and went to question Laurie, whom she found crying in the bathroom. Judy took one look at her daughter's tear-stained face and knew what had occurred. In the ensuing days, Judy confronted Tom and made arrangements to separate Laurie from him while trying to figure out what to do next. But before Judy reported him to the authorities, Laurie told a friend whose mother reported the abuse. The police subsequently arrested both parents and placed the children with Judy's parents.

To capture the intense emotional distress and turmoil of a mother discovering that her daughter is being abused by her husband, and the chaos that can ensue when the abuse becomes public, Judy's account in her own words follows:

JUDY: One night I got up in the middle of the night and I found him [Tom] by her room, and I asked him, what was going on, and he said that Laurie was having a nightmare and that he was waking her up. It sounded logical. Daddys do that. But I looked at her face and I saw fear. And I was sexually abused growing up.

MARCIA[1]: You were?

JUDY: Yes. And I knew it wasn't that he was waking her up, and I pulled her in the bathroom and Laurie told me that Daddy was touching her in places that he shouldn't be touching her. And when I got out of the bathroom with her, I opened the door to kick him out. He wouldn't leave. He slammed the door shut and pushed me against the wall and told me that he wasn't leaving, and if I called the cops that they would come and take the kids away from me because nobody would believe us because he works for the government—the cops would believe him,

---

[1]The therapist was Marcia Sheinberg. The team included Fiona True, Peter Fraenkel, and Sippio Small.

not us. I got really scared (*crying*). I didn't know what to do, and I guess—I don't even know—I was shocked and stunned and mortified that he would do this to my daughter, especially knowing that it happened to me.

MARCIA: That he knew it happened to you.

JUDY: And he knew how it hurt me that he would do this to her. I didn't know the extent of it until a couple of days later when Laurie asked me [at the table] if she could get pregnant. And I told her, what do you mean? I said, did you have—did he have intercourse with you? Laurie said yeah. Oh, my God. But he wouldn't leave me alone, you know? It was like he was always around and I didn't—you know, I was like, OK, I gotta get my head together, I gotta think. I was afraid. So what I did was I kept Laurie out of the house. My mom lives a few blocks away, and what I did was during the day after school I sent Laurie to my mom's, and when he was in bed, because he worked nights and he'd go to bed about seven, I let her come home and do her homework. She'd go to bed after her shower and then I'd stay up until he left for work, and then I would go to bed. And all I was waiting for was to call the cops when he wasn't around, so that he couldn't hurt us. Also, my dad has a heart condition, so I wanted him to go for his bypass, so that he would be OK, and then I would go stay with him and call the cops. Tom wouldn't know that I called, so that he couldn't hurt Laurie or me. What happened was Laurie told her friend, and the day that I was going to go stay with my parents, the cops came and they took us out of the house.

MARCIA: Both of—you and him?

JUDY: No, the kids. Then they put my kids in my parents' custody and they arrested me and they arrested him, because when the detective asked me if I knew what happened, I said I just found out 10 days ago. And I was, like, so relieved that they were there, that he would be out of the house (*begins to cry*) and that he wasn't going to hurt us. But I didn't know that I was in trouble because—I tried to protect the best I could, but I found out in court that he did sodomy to her, he had oral sex with her, and—and he was going into her room three times a week. And I don't know how he did this with me in the house sleeping and I didn't hear him. And Laurie didn't say anything because he told her that if she told me, that he would either kill her or I wouldn't believe her.

A PARENT'S DILEMMAS UPON DISCOVERY
OF ABUSE

Immediately upon learning of her daughter's abuse, Judy faced several difficult dilemmas. First, she was conflicted about whether to report Tom to the
authorities. She wanted to protect her daughter's physical and emotional
well-being, but for several reasons, Judy hoped to do this effectively without immediately reporting Tom. She didn't want to cause her ill father and
her mother additional stress. She worried about how her younger children
would react to the loss of their father, to whom they were very attached.
She wanted to figure out a way to explain the situation to them before having Tom removed from the home. Judy was also frightened about what Tom
might do if she reported him, because he had been so threatening when she
confronted him. And as a nonworking mother with three children, she also
worried about how the family would survive without his support if he went
to jail.

In addition, despite the tremendous sense of anger and betrayal she
felt toward Tom, and the upset she felt for her daughter, Judy also experienced the pull of her attachment toward him—feelings of love that were
uncomplicated just days earlier. Some background on their relationship
helps to explain her conflicting feelings. Judy became pregnant as a teenager, had her daughter, and continued to live with her parents, who supported both mother and child. Life was uneventful for Judy, and at times
lonely. Meeting Tom felt like a blessing. He was kind, extremely attentive,
and adored Laurie. He also had a good job and was enough of a take-charge
person that Judy felt secure leaving her parents to begin a new family. Judy
married Tom when Laurie was 6 years old. Judy was 24 at the time. She believed that with Tom, she had finally achieved her dream of creating her
own family, for Laurie as well as for herself. In quick succession, Judy and
Tom had two children. She came to trust Tom so much that she told him
her most troublesome secret: that she had been sexually abused by her
cousin. So for Tom to break this family apart by abusing Laurie and abusing
Judy's trust felt devastating and unimaginable. As is the case for many other
women, added to her turmoil was the reawakening of her own history of
abuse.

Tom's abuse of Laurie forced Judy into a situation in which any action
she took would affect the lives of all the people she loved, *who for the first
time had radically divergent and competing needs*. Yet Judy's attempt to balance
protecting Laurie, her other children, and her parents, and her need for
time to integrate the emotional and practical implications of the abuse led

her not to report Tom and resulted in her arrest on a charge of neglect. In Judy's words, this was a situation in which she felt "damned if you do, damned if you don't."

Therapeutic Choice Point: Whom to See First

It is in this context—one of confusion and emotional turmoil, family fragmentation, and involvement of the larger system, so poignantly described by Judy—that we typically meet the family. The first choice point for therapists is whom in the family to see first. Our approach is to meet with the mother alone before meeting with her child. This allows us to devote concentrated time to providing her with support, to addressing her concerns about engaging in treatment (without having to worry about how the child might experience hearing her concerns), and to gathering history. In addition, in the initial sessions alone with a mother, we not only elicit her version of the events surrounding the abuse but also communicate that we are interested in her total experience. In this way, we provide the mother with what is often her first opportunity to give voice to the complexity of her experience of the events, of her relationships, and of her sense of self in the aftermath of disclosure.

After meeting alone with Judy, we asked her to bring Laurie with her to the next session. She agreed to do so.

Therapeutic Choice Point: How Much to Focus Initially on the Abuse

Although we knew that Laurie had endured a long and possibly traumatic abuse, we also knew that Judy's recent arrest and the breakup of the family might have been equally traumatic—or at least might be more immediately salient for Laurie. Because we believe it is important from the outset to allow families to set the agenda for the session, our practice in this first family session is to state to mother and daughter our understanding that they have come because the child was abused (and here we state by whom). We state that although we certainly expect to be talking about what happened, we are also interested in family members' present struggles (which may be more immediately pressing for them). We encourage them to talk about whatever they would like to bring up. Typically, they choose first to discuss the events surrounding disclosure and current related issues.

In the initial meeting with Judy and Laurie we learned that they were having a rather difficult time with each other. Judy found Laurie "fresh," and Laurie found herself getting angry with her mother and, despite herself, saying mean things.

MARCIA: Your mom told me what happened from the time that you told her about your stepdad, and though I think it is something we will talk about in the future, I am interested in how things have been for you since you've been separated from your mom and stepdad?

LAURIE: It's been a little upsetting. We're not home with my mom. All of us want to be home with my mom, me and my brothers.

MARCIA: So you're all living there with your grandma and grandpa? How is it?

LAURIE: We always yell at each other . . . because sometimes I don't want to do what they want me to do, and sometimes I'm too lazy to get up (*laughs*).

MARCIA: So you give them a bit of a hard time? (*Laurie nods.*) Do you give your mom a hard time or just your grandparents?

LAURIE: I give my mom a hard time, too, sometimes (*laughs*).

There was further discussion about how Laurie behaved, particularly that she had a bad temper and, according to her mother, "a big mouth." Judy was clearly angry with Laurie and believed that she was uncooperative with her as well as her grandparents. According to Judy, this behavior had worsened. For her part, Laurie described her angry and defiant behavior, particularly with her mother, as "slips," saying, "I don't know why, but this nastiness just slips out." The need for her mother, and her anger at her mother, were not expressed directly in language, but in verbal action. Unfortunately, it seemed that Laurie's actions resulted in Judy's anger toward her instead of the comfort she needed so much.

As will be illustrated in upcoming vignettes from this therapy, the two ideas that kept Laurie from speaking to her mother and got acted out in her anger were her belief that Judy should have checked on her at night, so that she would have discovered Tom in Laurie's bed, and that Judy was angry with her for telling a friend about the abuse, which led to intervention by child welfare and the breakup of the family. Laurie may have believed that telling her mother either of these thoughts risked evoking Judy's anger or even rejection. Again, the dilemma for Laurie was that although she wanted to be closer to her mother, she feared that what she had to say could result in the loss of Judy's love.

Therapeutic Choice Point: How to Handle a Mother's Anger at Her Daughter

As we heard Judy and Laurie talk about their conflicts, we realized that Judy did harbor anger toward Laurie. We then faced a choice point— whether to explore Judy's anger in this first session with Laurie or find another time to do so, possibly first in a session with Judy alone. On the one hand, therapy should invite family members to express the full range of their feelings about one another. Furthermore, if Judy continued to be angry and critical, she would not be able to give Laurie the comfort and support that she needed more than ever. And if Laurie experienced Judy's anger toward her, she might believe that it originated not from her behaving disobediently, but more from how her mother felt about the abuse and/or its disclosure. Additionally, Laurie might also be angry with her mother for not protecting her and be afraid to express these feelings openly. Their fights over Laurie not cleaning up after herself, talking back, and being generally uncooperative might be easier to manage than confronting some aspects of their feelings about one another concerning the abuse.

On the other hand, the emotional turmoil surrounding the abuse, Laurie's emotional vulnerability as a result of the trauma, and her need for parental support in the aftermath suggested that we needed to help Judy find the balance between expressing anger and frustration with Laurie and modulating these feelings in the interest of reconnecting with and supporting her. For these latter reasons, we decided that strengthening the connection between Judy and Laurie needed to precede further discussion of Judy's anger toward her daughter. The following exchange between Marcia and Judy in Laurie's presence helps turn a criticism into a positive description.

MARCIA: Are you different from your daughter in this way [referring to "big mouth"]?

JUDY: I let people hurt me and hurt me, and I let it build up.

MARCIA: And what do you do after it's built up?

JUDY: Then I blow up and I'll yell, and then I won't take it anymore. [She offers a recent example of how she confronted a woman who had been gossiping about her. Marcia responds by inquiring about how her response is different from what Laurie's would be in that situation.] Laurie will tell you right there and then.

MARCIA: Laurie doesn't let it build?

JUDY: No. No. Laurie will tell you where it's at.

MARCIA: Do you like that quality in your daughter?

JUDY: Yes. Yes, because I don't think that Laurie will ever take what I take, and I'm learning not to take it anymore, because it's not fair that people can do that to you. I always say they play head games with you, and I'm not going to let people do that.

The mood in the room shifted almost palpably as mother and daughter connected through discussion of the positive side of a quality Laurie possessed that at times emerged in a form that angered her mother. In this more accepting atmosphere, Laurie's relational struggles and confusions began to unfold.

AN ABUSED CHILD'S CONFLICTUAL FEELINGS

One source of Laurie's confusion concerned her conflicting feelings about Tom. On the one hand, Laurie received empathy as the victim of her stepfather's abuse. Her upset and angry feelings were validated by her family, friends, and professionals. On the other hand, she secretly had positive feelings toward him. Additionally, Laurie was repeatedly reassured by others that he was responsible for what happened, but she also secretly believed that she was responsible. On the one hand are the feelings that Laurie believed were acceptable; on the other were the shameful and therefore secret feelings. The following exchange with Laurie alone came after a rather lengthy description by mother and daughter of a recent time in court, in which the outcome was that the children could not yet return to their mother. Both mother and daughter expressed their upset and anger over the separation.

Following further discussion between mother and daughter about their separation, in an individual session with Laurie, Marcia asked about the separation from Tom.

MARCIA: Can I ask you a hard question?

LAURIE: OK.

MARCIA: Do you miss Tom?

LAURIE: I do miss him a little 'cause he was there when I got glass in my hand, a splinter in my finger, and when I had to go to the hospital 'cause I—I was rollerblading and I fell on my side and he brought me to the hospital. So he was there more times than my father was and I do miss him a little. He took me to get ice cream, he bought me stuff, and he was really nice. Like, he would watch movies with me and my mom, and he would really watch any kind of movies. He'd watch movies that are sad, movies that people die in, and horror movies—well, he really [never] liked horror movies but I always watched them, so he would watch them with me.

MARCIA: So he really did stuff with you like that.

LAURIE: Mm hmm.

Again, because in conversations with the professional community, Laurie's stepfather had only been described as abusive, and other descriptions of him were absent, Laurie may have felt that it was wrong to have any positive feelings toward him. The conflict for her centered not only on whether to state the feelings but also, on a more fundamental level, whether even to have them. In other words, she may have had to deny these feelings to herself. When Marcia asked Laurie if she missed Tom, she conveyed that it was OK to express positive as well as negative feelings toward him. Conveying this with her mother present made it clear that Laurie need not keep her positive feelings toward Tom a secret.

FOLLOWING THE CHILD'S LEAD

When the child begins to talk about the abuse, we follow her lead. We make it clear that she can talk about it as much or as little as she'd like. We also let her choose with whom she'd like to begin talking about it—in the family session with her mother, or with the therapist alone. As most children do, Laurie chose to talk for the first time about the abuse alone with the therapist. Giving the child the choice of how much and with whom to speak about the abuse is one of the first of many moments throughout the therapy in which we provide the child with the opportunity to enhance her sense of agency and control—a sense that was violated by the person who offended.

Like most children, Laurie was reluctant to speak about the abuse initially, and so we offered her an explanation of why we felt it was important to speak about it; then, as described earlier, we gave her the option to talk with us about it or not. Note that the rationale we gave Laurie for talking about her abuse experiences has two elements: an internal, intrapsychic one and a relational one.

MARCIA: I know that it's very hard to talk about. So I think what I want to explain to you is why I think it's important to talk about it, and then you can decide if you are willing to talk and how much.

LAURIE: OK.

MARCIA: I think when it stays a secret between you and Tom, and even though it is not happening now, you may feel that only he knows some things about you, and this may keep you from feeling completely good about yourself. The other reason is that I think the more you talk about it, and the different feelings you had, the more you will be able to remember without feeling as upset as you do now. So I thought that if you're willing, we'd begin a little bit today. We'll go slowly, and you'll actually tell me about specifically what happened and when it started, what you remember. What do you think about that?

LAURIE: OK. But sometimes it's a little hard for me to explain what happened.

MARCIA: What makes it hard?

LAURIE: It's just what he did to me makes me all upset . . .

MARCIA: Of course.

LAURIE: . . . and it's, like, when I had to go to the place that night when they took me out of my house, I had to explain it about five times or something. I had to explain it a lot of times, explain it to two people a lot of times. Then someone else would come in and I would have to explain it to her.

MARCIA: I think that what they were trying to do was get the evidence so that they could arrest Tom. What we will do that I think might be different is to talk more about what it felt like for you.

After a few moments of quiet, Laurie began to describe her experience of the abuse.

LAURIE: I was just crying. I put a pillow over my head. Then I wouldn't see him. I put a pillow over my head and made believe I was sleeping, or just closed my eyes and tears came down my eyes, and . . . I put a whole bunch of covers on me, and I just wrapped them around me . . . just wrapped them around me and just made believe that he couldn't touch me because I was wrapped around so many blankets. But he would just touch me and then when he was done, he would just leave and it seemed all better the next morning. He would never talk about it.

As Laurie continued her description, she included how she questioned her own culpability.

MARCIA: Help me understand more about why you blamed yourself when your stepfather, Tom, came into the room and did this to you. Why did you blame yourself?

LAURIE: Because I was wearing T-shirts, not short but long T-shirts, and I would kind of think maybe he thought that I was trying to tell him something, but I wasn't. But I thought that maybe I was doing something I didn't know I was telling him. I was just thinking about different things every time, and it would just be a whole bunch of things in my head.

MARCIA: Right. What other things?

LAURIE: Um, that—I was kind of a little pretty. I was hoping that I'd be ugly so that he wouldn't do it anymore to me. Sometimes I prayed let me be ugly tonight. Let me just be ugly just for tonight, and then tomorrow I'll be so pretty. And it would never happen. I'll always be the same person, and I think maybe I was too pretty, maybe I was not acting my age. I was, like, being older than I was supposed to. Maybe he thought I was giving him some ideas.

We can see how confusing the experience is for a child—how Laurie tried to stop the abuse, or at least, psychologically shelter herself from it, and how she repeatedly experienced her powerlessness. Yet, Laurie still wondered if she was responsible. In the following session Laurie elaborated her feelings:

MARCIA: Did you have any thoughts about our last session?

LAURIE: No, it's just that it's hard for me to talk a little more about it. When I went home, I just started thinking about it, and when I went to bed I cried 'cause it just hurts me. And I was thinking in the car when we were coming here, when am I going to wake up from this nightmare, you know?

MARCIA: And what was the answer you gave yourself to that question?

LAURIE: Nothing (*laughs*). I just started listening to music again.

MARCIA: To get your mind off it?

LAURIE: Yeah.

MARCIA: Well that's good. Should I tell you again why I think it's important that we talk about it?

LAURIE: No, that's OK. I think I know why.

MARCIA: Why, in your mind?

LAURIE: Because, um, sometimes when you talk about it, it doesn't hurt as much as when it is inside, and that it's not a secret anymore 'cause other people know.

MARCIA: So should we continue to talk about it?

LAURIE: Yes. You ask me a question.

MARCIA: OK. When you were crying, what were you thinking about or feeling?

LAURIE: I was feeling upset that I trusted him, and I thought he was a real father to me. Also, it was just so strange that one day everything was OK and the next day it's, like, our family broke. I was just lying there trying to sleep but I couldn't. And I was trying to think of different things. The TV was on and I was watching the news, but I couldn't, I was just so upset.

MARCIA: Were you thinking about actual things that he did to you or more about the idea of the family being broken?

LAURIE: What he did to me.

MARCIA: Were you picturing it?

LAURIE: Yeah. It's been happening a lot of times now. Sometimes when I'm all right in class, I can do my work, I talk to my friends, I pass letters back and forth around, and then I just get a strange thing that I see— what happened to me—and I just get all upset.

MARCIA: What do you actually see?

LAURIE: I see him touching me, and just . . .

MARCIA: Can you tell me the picture you see in detail?

LAURIE: Him putting his private part into me, touching my leg, and then, uh, and then, like, he would just leave and the picture would be gone. But I would always get the same picture back again and again.

MARCIA: Did he say anything to you?

LAURIE: Not a lot of times. Sometimes I would try to push him off of me, but it—it was too hard so—and I couldn't. He told me not to tell my mother 'cause I would have been taken away from her, and I would never see my mother ever again. And he threatened me. If I told my mother, when he comes out of jail, he would kill me.

AN ABUSED CHILD'S DILEMMA: TO TELL OR NOT TO TELL

Laurie's account of Tom's threats about what would happen to her if she told anyone about the sexual abuse describes well the forces that caused her, as well as other children in this situation, a dilemma over disclosure. On the one hand, children want the protection from the nonoffending parent that telling could bring, yet are fearful that what they will receive is disbelief and more harm.

Laurie's Fear of Retaliation

Marcia shifts the focus of the session to the present.

MARCIA: Are you scared now of his coming to get you?

LAURIE: A little. Sometimes in the night I see him. I dreamt that my mother said we were all going to be a family again, and then I saw Tom take out a gun, and I ran. He shot me, and I was on the ground covered with blood, dead.

Therapeutic Choice Point: Whether to Widen the Relational Focus

Laurie's dream was a clear expression of her fear that her mother would reunite with Tom and that she would not be protected from his anger. At this point, we had different therapeutic choices. One was to elaborate Laurie's fears of Tom; another, to broaden the lens to include Laurie's perception of her mother's feelings about Tom.

Because Laurie's fears of Tom were grounded in actual threats he made to her, these were quite understandable. Less clear was why, as the dream suggested, Laurie worried that her mother would return to him despite the abuse. Since this may have been more difficult to articulate, Marcia, by asking Laurie for her ideas about her mother's attachment to Tom, helped Laurie put her concerns into words.

MARCIA: That sounds like a frightening and very upsetting dream. I'm wondering, do you think in some way that your mother misses Tom?

LAURIE: I think a little 'cause sometimes when he was a nice man, my mom loves him for that and for my brothers. But I think that my mom's happy that we got the bad guy out of the house 'cause I think she would think of her kids first, and that's the truth 'cause I remember when I was in third grade, my mom walked me to school and she said that her children come first and her husband comes second. So my mom's probably happy that he's out. And, she's probably worried that when I am a teenager, he would do it again to me.

MARCIA: Laurie, would you like to tell your mother about the dream?

LAURIE: I was going to tell her about my dream and say I'm a little scared, 'cause sometimes I do think about it—that I'll walk out of my house and he's right there and he takes me away and he just kills me. That's what I think of sometimes. One day I sat and I wrote down things to tell my mom about, like my dream, but I ripped up the paper into, like, a hundred pieces and just threw it out.

MARCIA: Why, Laurie?

LAURIE: 'Cause it's hard for me to talk to my mom about Tom.

MARCIA: If you had given her the paper, what would you want your mother to say to you that would make you feel better?

LAURIE: That she wouldn't go back with him. But she'll probably say that he won't come and do something to me, that she'll keep me safe.

MARCIA: What about going back with him?

LAURIE: She wouldn't, 'cause she said to me that she wouldn't go back with him, that her life right now is just gonna be me and my brothers.

MARCIA: It seems that the dream is different, that your mom is back with him.

Therapeutic Choice Point: When to State What the Client Has Left Unspoken

One critical choice point in all therapy is when to state your hunch about feelings that the client has not directly articulated. The choice is between sticking to the content of what the client is saying or "pushing it" a little further and, if pushing it, how to do this sensitively and not leave the client more upset than before.

For instance, we believed that Laurie was struggling with her fear that Judy might reunite with Tom, and that as much as Laurie tried to reassure herself by reminding herself that Judy had said that her children come first, the dream spoke another truth. Therefore, Marcia chose to articulate a possible basis for Laurie's worry to see if it resonated for her. Marcia's tone and language were speculative, so that it was clearly Marcia's thought about a thought that Laurie might have but had not yet named. In naming Laurie's possible concern, Marcia opened the door for Laurie to talk about an even more important, unarticulated belief—that her mother knew about the abuse while it was occurring and didn't choose to protect her.

MARCIA: Do you think it's possible that one of the reasons you might have had the dream is because you know she misses parts of Tom—the good parts? (*Laurie nods.*) So maybe you think if she misses those parts of him, maybe she would decide to go back and that you would not be protected again?

LAURIE: Yeah. She saw him around my room a couple of times, but my mom didn't catch on.

MARCIA: Do you think she should have?

LAURIE: Yeah, I think she should have—'cause my mom did ask me a couple of times if anyone is touching me . . .

MARCIA: So she was suspicious?

LAURIE: Yeah. I guess she was just wondering if anything's going on, but I would always lie, and it was hard for me to lie to her.

MARCIA: I bet. I bet it was.

LAURIE: And I always wanted to tell her. Sometimes I'd just say, "MA!" And she'd say what? And—'cause I wanted to tell her—but I would say never mind.

MARCIA: So does a part of you feel like she should have figured it out?

LAURIE: Yeah.

MARCIA: And protected you? (*Laurie nods yes.*) Am I putting words in your mouth or is that what you feel?

LAURIE: No. That's how I feel.

MARCIA: And because you're very close to your mother and you feel very protective toward her, is it hard for you to recognize that you feel that toward her at the same time that you love her?

LAURIE: Yeah.

MARCIA: Could you explain to me how that works for you?

LAURIE: 'Cause I'm the closest one to my mom, and I thought she would protect me. I thought she would probably get up at night to see if he's in my room or something.

MARCIA: She should have checked?

LAURIE: Yeah, but my mom said that probably the reason why she didn't wake up is 'cause she trusted Tom. And that's the reason why I trusted him, too, but now the trust is gone from him, 'cause I don't trust him ever.

MARCIA: Do you think your mom is convinced that he's not to be trusted? Ever?

LAURIE: I don't think my mom trusts him anymore. I don't think my mom will ever trust him anymore, and I don't—and the truth is, I don't think my mom would go back with him.

MARCIA: Well, my guess is that the dream says that you are still anxious. You know what anxious means? Like nervous, worried. That even though in one way you can tell yourself that your mother's not going to go back with him, in some way it makes you worry because . . .

LAURIE: She still has little parts of her that love him.

MARCIA: Well, would it help if you and your mom talked about this openly?

LAURIE: It would kind of help.

MARCIA: How should we do it? You'll talk to her and I'll just help you? Not that you need help, but . . .

LAURIE: Can you talk to her for me (laughs)?

MARCIA: Want me to talk to her for you?

LAURIE: Yeah. 'Cause I get a little nervous when I talk—like, I can't really talk to my mom about a lot of stuff 'cause I get nervous.

Therapeutic Choice Point: Whether and How to Link Individual and Family Sessions

As can be seen, individual sessions allow abused children to discuss challenging feelings and beliefs about themselves, the person who offended, and the nonoffending parent in a manner that might be difficult if the nonoffending parent were present.

After a rather full exploration of Laurie's different feelings about loyalty, attachment, and protection, Marcia engaged her in a Decision Dialogue to decide how to bring the new information and insights back to her mother in a family session. Although we offered Laurie the privacy she needed to explore the complexity of her feelings, Judy was her ongoing resource for healing. As Laurie gets older, the abuse experience will have different meanings, and it is critical that she can turn toward Judy and trust her with any of the feelings she may experience connected to the abuse. In the following excerpt from a session with Laurie and Judy, the fears and concerns that Laurie expressed in the individual session were first communicated to her mother in a family session.

MARCIA: We were talking about a dream Laurie had in which you take Tom back to live with you. And that even though you said your children come first, and you're not going to go back with him, a part of her knows there's a part of you that loves certain parts of him, and that maybe in the future, you would go back with him, and that would make her feel—that makes her feel, we think, a little anxious, even though Laurie says she knows you're not going to.

LAURIE: And don't forget the one with the shooting.

MARCIA: Could you tell?

LAURIE: One day I saw you and—you and Tom—and you turned around and said that it's OK, we'll all be a family again, and then I saw him pull out a gun and he—I was running and he shot me, and I was—and I was on the floor with blood all over me, and I was dead.

JUDY (*pausing, then speaking emphatically and reassuringly*): Let me just tell you, I will never get back together with Tom, because of what he did to you and to us. He destroyed any type of love that anybody could ever have. So you don't ever have to worry about that, OK? When someone does something like that, they're sick. And he's going to be away a very, very, very long time, OK? So you don't have to worry. The part of Tom that I loved, like I said, isn't who Tom is now, OK? So that's—that's gone, that's over with. So you don't ever have to be worried that I would ever even consider taking him back, OK?

LAURIE: Thank you (*tears streaming down her face*).

MARCIA: (*to Laurie*) What are the tears? What are you feeling?

LAURIE: 'Cause I'm talking to her face-to-face.

MARCIA: And what makes you cry when you talk to your mom face to face?

LAURIE: I don't know, it's just strange, 'cause I really don't talk to my mom about Tom a lot (*cries*).

JUDY: Oh, baby. I know. It's OK. But I love you. It's OK to be afraid, but just don't ever doubt that he would ever come back, OK? OK? He can never, ever, ever, ever, ever, ever, ever hurt you again, OK? OK? I promise. (*Judy gets up and takes her daughter in her arms, holds her and strokes her hair as Laurie sobs.*)

A CHILD'S TURMOIL: WHETHER TO EXPRESS NEGATIVE FEELINGS TOWARD THE NONOFFENDING PARENT

As this session illustrates, once Laurie became more aware and articulate about her feelings of anger, hurt, fear, and disappointment toward Judy, she faced the dilemma of whether to share these feelings with her.

Once again, the practice of including a Decision Dialogue at the end of each individual session with Laurie allowed us to discuss openly her concerns about expressing feelings to her mother, and to come up with a plan about how to do this in a way that would not further traumatize her. At first, as did Laurie, children often ask the therapist to convey their feelings to the parent. As therapy progresses and the child has an increasing number of positive experiences expressing her feelings and concerns to her parent, she becomes increasingly comfortable speaking about these feelings and concerns directly.

In the case of Laurie, we believed Judy would be responsive and not critical of her, and we encouraged Laurie to bring up her concerns in a meeting with her mother. If the child is really scared to talk with the parent, even if we have perceived the parent to be responsive, we meet with the parent first to explore the child's concerns about speaking.

As much as Laurie tried to reassure herself that her mother would not again live with Tom, she needed to hear it directly from Judy. We also believe that Laurie sensed her mother's ambivalence and that it needed to be addressed further with Judy. Yet, prior to this session, Laurie could not speak with her mother directly. Throughout the remaining sessions, we built on this positive experience Laurie had in speaking with her mother, so as to encourage Laurie to bring up other concerns, including her anger that

Judy did not report the abuse immediately to the police, and the fear that she secretly blamed Laurie for disclosing the abuse to a friend.

Whom you can talk to and what you can talk about were for Laurie recurring themes that, if unaddressed, might have left her vulnerable in the future by encouraging her to keep as secrets painful or dangerous experiences, rather than seeking out a protective other. Likewise, if we had not given Judy ample opportunity to discuss her feelings about Tom, her unprocessed attachment could have made Laurie's fears a reality.

DUAL DILEMMAS FOR THERAPIST AND PARENT: WHETHER AND HOW TO ADDRESS ATTACHMENT TO AN ABUSIVE PARTNER

Nonoffending parents often feel quite ashamed of their continued emotional attachment to the offending partner. As a result, therapists often feel reluctant to ask questions about this attachment, and parents feel reluctant to bring it up.

In addition, as we noted earlier, because the referral for therapy is based on the child's having been abused, therapists have a tendency to relate to nonoffending parents only in their role as the child's mother. Their other identities can too easily be ignored in the face of the abuse perpetrated by her husband or partner. Yet these women continue to have needs that, until recently, had been fulfilled by their partners. It is easy to understand that they would feel judged negatively for continued longings for their partners, and would be reluctant to express them. Laurie recognized Judy's continued attachment to Tom, an awareness first revealed by the content of her fearful dream.

In the following dialogue, Marcia encourages Judy to articulate the many feelings she has about Tom. The more freely she can share all her feelings, the clearer she will be and the more able to make a sound assessment of her relationship with him.

MARCIA: I want to give you space in here because, besides being a mother, you are a wife, and this must be hard.

JUDY: You know, I loved him so much. We were good together. We had a good relationship. He was my best friend (*begins to cry*). And it's hard not being able to—to talk to him about how I'm feeling. I mean, every—every—we did everything together, not because we had to but we just enjoyed it. Like *Cheers*, he loved *Cheers*. I used to come home. My God, I used to complain. Now, every week I put *Cheers* on—to make me feel like I'm with him a little bit. And then I say to myself, no, it's wrong. You're not supposed to have feelings like that. Look what he did to Laurie, look what he did to us. And then there is a little part of me that says, "Yes, he did do that, and yes, he's being punished, but you can still love him."

MARCIA: Mm hm. And miss him. You miss him.

JUDY: And it breaks my heart with the babies because they're constantly asking for him. You know, in his desk drawer, I didn't clean that part out yet, and there is his picture, and they look at it and they kiss him. They ask if he's coming home. It just hurts. You know, I just want—I just—I don't know. I mean, I say to myself, I forgave my cousin and I still love my cousin. Why can't—if he gets help and it's guaranteed—although there are never any guarantees in life, but why can't I be with him? Not them, but me, myself, on a one-to-one basis. Never let him come home—do you know what I'm saying? Like, just talk to him (*she cries*).

MARCIA: So you're just thinking about how you could do that or whether you could do that.

JUDY: Right, right. And you know, I would never—I mean, there would always be a part of me that would never trust him with my kids. But I also—there is another part of me that's really sad they'll never know him. I look through the photo albums and I see when I had the kids and him in the delivery room with me. It's just sad.

MARCIA: It is sad. It is sad. Sad for the kids and sad for you. It sounds like—from the time that you wanted to go to the jail and tell him off—that was one side of your feelings, your rage and anger, but it sounds like now . . .

JUDY: I still want to tell him off, and tell him, "Why did you do this? Because we had everything anybody in life wants. You have a good marriage, you have a nice relationship, you have decent money, you have a beautiful house, beautiful family, everybody is healthy. You have everything, a job that you're proud of, you're going to school. Why did you destroy that?"

MARCIA: It feels like it doesn't make sense as you remember all the good things.

JUDY: Exactly. Tom was the only person I ever knew who could tell by looking at me, by hearing my voice, how I felt. You know, I miss that. I miss the hugs (*cries*). I'm sorry.

MARCIA: That's OK, that's OK (*hands Judy a box of tissues*).

JUDY: You know, even when he wrote his resignation letter for work, he put in it that I'm to get everything. All the money and everything. So another part of me is saying, "The louse really messed up. Look what he did." Yet he's still trying to take care of us, you know? I just don't understand why . . .

MARCIA: He did it?

JUDY: Yeah. I just—I don't—I can't figure it out. Last night the VCR broke. I don't know what happened. It got messed up. Laurie was mad because I couldn't tape her show. So I'm sitting there and I'm playing with it, and she says, "I wish Tom was here." And I said, "I wish so too, because this would have never broke."

MARCIA: It's nice that you can say that to each other. Those are the parts of him you miss, you really miss.

JUDY: Yeah.

MARCIA: And it's nice that she could say it and then you could say it. Well, you're in a tough, tough spot. You really are. Because there are parts of you that really want him, and you don't understand what this is about, why he's been like this. I think he has some attraction to young girls. I don't know, because I don't know him. But I think the way you're trying to put it together is to say, "OK, if this is an illness he has and he can get cured, then maybe in the future I can have a relationship with him."

JUDY: Right, but not with the children.

MARCIA: I think it's hard for you to accept this ending in which he's out of your life for good, without even understanding why he did what he did. There is no closure.

JUDY: Exactly. Exactly. Yet I don't think I could ever trust him again.

At this time, it is clear that Judy misses her previous life and struggles to make sense of her husband's betrayal. She is distinguishing between her needs as a woman and her responsibilities as a parent. In subsequent sessions, she begins to distinguish between wanting a partner and wanting Tom. By freely sharing her feelings of shame, she begins to relate more and more to her angry feelings, and it is in this context of engaging the full and complex range of her interior life that Judy finds a stronger voice. She begins to take pleasure in her own competence. While she struggles financially, and eventually begins to date, she shares with us how she quickly extricates herself from situations that are not in her best interest. She is more discriminating in her friendships.

THERAPEUTIC CHOICE POINT: HOW TO QUESTION APPROACHES TO PARENTING

Parents often hold strong beliefs about the adequacy of their parenting, and these beliefs are usually tied to their families and cultures of origin. Either they replicate approaches they experienced as children or attempt to parent differently than they were parented. However, sometimes parents repeat approaches they did not like, or they feel unable to enact new patterns. Sometimes they are not aware of the connection between what they experienced as children and how they are parenting. In any case, addressing parenting styles must be done respectfully.

As therapy with Judy and Laurie continued, we were aware that Judy tended to issue orders to Laurie, and that Laurie tended more often to act out her feelings than to discuss them. Because Judy felt so criticized about her parenting by others, we recognized that intervening in this area could be quite delicate. Yet we strongly believed that Laurie needed to feel she could talk with her mother. Although we have already described the different ways we encouraged this (through opening up difficult topics), we had not yet called into question more directly Judy's style of communicating with Laurie. We chose to do so at this point in the therapy, first, because it had persisted despite other changes, and second, because we believed that Judy had come to feel very accepted and valued by us.

One of the most informative and least threatening ways we have found to initiate discussion about parenting is first to ask parents about their own childhood experiences with their parents, and what they preferred or did not like about their parents' approach. Marcia asked Judy about the way she was mothered, and learned that Judy never spoke with her mother about anything intimate. When Marcia asked more about this, including what Judy thought might have been her mother's response if Judy had spoken, she said her mother would have been critical. When Marcia asked how Judy imagined her life would have been different had her mother been more accepting, Judy didn't miss a beat in exclaiming that everything would have been different: She would have had confidence to continue her education; she would have chosen different men. After both discussing the way Judy remembered her relationship with her mother and considering a different kind of mother–daughter relationship, it was an easy transition for Marcia to ask Judy to consider how she might change the legacy of the past by mothering Laurie differently.

A New Meaning of Mothering

When Laurie and Judy returned for the next session, both described a new experience together. They had spent time together in a relaxing way, talking, watching television, and snacking. Judy described it as their being more like friends than mother and daughter. As this was explored, Judy came to speak about it as being a "more relaxed mother." To her surprise, she even found herself suggesting to her own mother that she might just visit them and not worry so much about everything being neat and tidy. And, as Judy began defining mothering in new ways, Laurie seemed pleased and more able to confide in her mother.

A significant change in Laurie had also taken place. Previously, she had shared the thought that she was sure she was going to have a baby when she became a teenager. Having shared this belief with her mother, Judy and Laurie talked over the notion that because Judy gave birth to Laurie when she was a teenager, this did not mean that Laurie was destined to do the same. In addition, with some input from us, they had discussed the possibility that Laurie herself missed being the youngest child and that the image of having a baby represented her own wish to be babied a bit by her mother. Laurie—who previously said the belief that she would have a child as a teen was not experienced as just a thought but as a *feeling in her body*—was surprised that she now believed she would become a mother only when she was in her late twenties or early thirties.

Therapeutic Choice Point: Whether and How to Involve the Person Who Offended

One of the trickiest, and most contentious issues in the literature on treatment of sexually abused children is whether to involve the person who offended in treatment, and if so, how. In an upcoming chapter, we describe in detail our approach to working directly with family members who offend and engaging them in family sessions. Here, we address the issue of whether and how to engage the offending family member in treatment when he will not be physically present in the treatment—whether because he is incarcerated, there is a legal injunction for him not to see the child, or the nonoffending parent or child refuses any further proximal contact with him. The usual reason for engaging an offending family member under such circumstances is to help clarify for the child that he, and not she, was responsible for the abuse.

The need for this in working with Laurie became apparent in an individual session with her following the session in which she so clearly had difficulty talking directly with her mother. In this session, we learned that she was inhibited by her belief that her mother held her responsible in part for the abuse. We also learned that Laurie held herself responsible. This knowledge allowed us to move in two directions that helped to free Laurie from this self-incrimination: (1) to have a session with mother and daughter in which the issue of "blame" was fully explored, and (2) to have the stepfather, with the therapist as an intermediary, write a letter in which he took complete responsibility for the abuse. The details of how to arrange this "apology" letter are described in Chapter 7. For Laurie, as well as for the other abused children with whom we work, having both parents be very clear that it is not the child's "fault," regardless of the circumstances, is enormously relieving. Time and time again, we find that children want to hear it from the person who abused them.

THE LARGER SYSTEM: SHOULD THE THERAPIST MAINTAIN A STANCE OF NEUTRALITY OR ACT AS AN ADVOCATE?

As with many of the families we see, various court-related personnel (the child's court-appointed lawyer, the district attorney, the nonoffending parent's lawyer, the judge) often request not only reports on treatment and recommendations about visitation, but also that we, at times, advocate a particular decision. Because the family knows this, it puts the therapy at risk of becoming inauthentic; that is, the adults act in a way that they think we would want, and in the worse-case scenario, instruct their children as to how to behave and what to say and not say. We can even appreciate the impetus for this by recalling how Judy was refused the return of her children at one point because Laurie's court-appointed guardian reported that, in a private meeting, Laurie had expressed anger toward her mother. On the one hand, if you choose to respond to larger system requests, the family knows that you can intervene to their perceived gain or detriment using information gathered in sessions, and this certainly may affect how family members relate to you.

On the other hand, if you choose to remain "neutral"—not to respond to larger system requests or to advocate for the family, this inactivity may permit terrible injustices to take place that damage the abused child and her siblings. In fact, the stance of "neutrality" is a misnomer, because it is a strong position in favor of believing that the legal system is the appropriate avenue for determining issues of reunification and visitation. However, if you do make a recommendation based on your knowledge of the family, it may not always be one the family desires.

In Chapter 4, we discuss how to navigate these dilemmas through a collaborative process with the family. In terms of our work with Laurie's family, we believed that though Judy was ambivalent about reporting Tom, to arrest her and to remove the children was a terribly misguided action. Given the young ages of the other children and the abrupt way they were separated from both parents, the disruption and pain caused by this legal intervention was enormous.

Therefore, we decided to intervene without being asked to do so. First, we invited Laurie's siblings to participate in some play sessions and observed them individually and together with their mother. Based on our observations of the children and our early sessions with Judy and Laurie, we offered to write a letter to the court stating why we believed the children needed to be home with their mother. We stated that we understood that the court's intention was to safeguard the welfare of the children, and that we shared that concern. However, we then suggested that the best protection for both the children's physical safety and emotional well-being was to return them to their mother and their home. In addition to this letter, when the court requested as part of the return that Judy enroll in a parenting skills course, we offered to supply the parenting information as part of our therapy and to report as required on her progress. And by involving Judy in a process of coauthoring these reports, what began for her as an invasive, disempowering experience became another opportunity to increase her sense of competence and personal agency.

Therapeutic Choice Point: When to Terminate Therapy

During 6 months of therapy, Laurie progressed a great deal in her recovery from abuse. At the beginning of treatment, she described intrusive thoughts, sexual preoccupations, difficulty in talking with her mother about the abuse, and feelings of responsibility for what had occurred. Six months later, she rarely experienced these symptoms, self-blaming thoughts, or difficulties communicating with her mother. Laurie herself said she did not think she needed therapy any longer, and from our perspective, to continue treatment at this point, we risked creating topics or looking for material. Judy, however, wanted to continue to come in, but perhaps on a less frequent basis. Her troubles at this time had more to do with survival issues, since the amount of money issued to her by public assistance was inadequate to sustain her family.

We responded to the idea of termination by suggesting that, for the following year, unless the family requested additional sessions, we would continue to see family members every 2 months. We typically suggest periodic sessions over time rather than a definite end to treatment, so as to encourage families to use us as a resource as they continue to face the challenges of life following disclosure. These challenges include adjustment to not having the person who offended in the family's life at all, or in the same way as before. When the person who offended is a father or other adult providing a substantial percentage of the family's income, as in the case of Tom, the family may face drastic economic challenges that require a change of lifestyle, address, schools, and so on. Family members may also need occasional support to sustain new patterns of relating to one another. Although we could simply terminate and suggest to family members that they call us if they need to, we find that it is comforting for families to know that they have set, future appointments.

Chapter Three

Core Perspectives

In this chapter, we describe the theories and general practices that guide our work with sexually abused children and their families. Building on ideas originally described by Sheinberg (1992), we discuss how we have drawn from social constructionist, feminist, and systems thinking to create the *relational* approach. As we describe, the relational approach is not a new theory, but rather can be viewed as a conceptual "umbrella" that links the three component theories in a manner that expands therapeutic possibilities.

After outlining which ideas and practices we draw from each source theory, we briefly review the key differences and tensions among them. We describe how we use these tensions to view the family from different perspectives and to remain accountable to the different concerns highlighted by each perspective.

The relational approach does not fit neatly into one of the three categories currently used to describe approaches to psychotherapy integration—technical eclecticism (drawing techniques from theoretically different approaches without concern for their contrasting source premises), theoretical integration (formulating a "conceptual framework that synthesizes the best elements of two or more approaches"; Norcross & Newman, 1992, p. 11), and common factors (locating the common concepts among different theories; Lebow, 1997; Norcross & Newman, 1992). In actual practice, our approach represents a possible fourth type of integration: *theoretical eclecticism*

51

(Fraenkel & Pinsof, in press), also called a "multitheoretical" perspective. In theoretical eclecticism, different theories serve as different lenses that highlight different aspects of a situation or phenomenon. When layered one upon the other, these lenses or perspectives serve both to reinforce areas of agreement, to fill in for each other's oversights, and, through the tension of the disagreements among them, to act to correct one another's excesses.

As an important aside, we wish to note that despite our interest in theory, in our discussions about families, we avoid using professional and theory-based language and jargon, preferring instead to describe families in plain English. For instance, although we are influenced by the professional metaphor of "narrative" or "story" in thinking about the impact of incest upon families, and by the notion of a "triangle" in thinking about loyalty binds among a child, nonoffending parent, and the offending family member, we rarely refer to these technical terms, either when talking among ourselves or with families.

Our reasons for attempting to remain "close to the ground" in our thinking and talking about families are at least twofold. First, given the great variety of children, families, and circumstances we've seen, with wide differences in their composition (e.g., who's in the "family"), styles of interaction, strengths and resources, cultural backgrounds, and particular incest experiences, we have found that basing our work on a few simple premises allows us great flexibility to meet the needs of the whole range of families. Second, we discuss families in a language that is readily accessible to them. We talk directly with families to construct useful explanations of how the incest occurred, what its impact has been, and how change can occur. Because we regularly share our thinking with family members, we prefer to discuss them among ourselves in the same language that we use to talk *with* them. This practice keeps the families "in the room" with us, even when they're not physically there, and keeps us thinking, "What might the family say to these ideas?" In this way, we remain in a dialogue that respects and empowers families at all times.

IDEAS AND PRACTICES
FROM SOCIAL CONSTRUCTIONISM

From social constructionist therapies (see, e.g., Freedman & Combs, 1996; McNamee & Gergen, 1992; White, 1992; White & Epston, 1990; Zimmerman & Dickerson, 1994), we have adapted, with some important modifications, three core foci and ideas:

1. The power of problem narratives and the importance of strengths
2. Multiple perspectives
3. Both–and versus either–or thinking

The Power of Problem Narratives and the Importance of Strengths

Social constructionists highlight the importance of language and narrative (the accounts persons tell themselves and others, or that are told to them, about their experience) in defining the meanings of events, experiences, and interactions. Problem-focused language and narratives—descriptions and accounts of individuals and families that focus on their difficulties rather than their strengths and resources—come to restrain meaning and possibility, making change increasingly difficult. From this perspective, therapy needs to focus on building family strengths and resources.

For instance, over the years, women who were sexually abused as children changed their description of themselves from "victims" to "survivors." The intent of this change in language was to capture better the strengths such women experienced about themselves as they strove to overcome the impact of victimization. Although, historically, the use of the term "victim" had the important effect of recasting intrafamilial abuse and battering as acts of violence rather than as an assumed privilege of men within their homes, the shift to the term "survivor" was the next important step in empowering victimized women.

Similarly, we avoid the term "offender," and speak rather of the "person who offended." This language suggests that the man or boy is not wholly described by his offending act. Such language sets the stage for him to take greater responsibility, for it is that part of him that is not "the offender" that must acknowledge the offense and develop the empathy and self-control that enables him to prevent abusive actions in the future.

The narrative metaphor (Freedman & Combs, 1996; Zimmerman & Dickerson, 1994; White & Epston, 1990) is essential to our notion of the incest experience as a "story of shame" that often dominates and obliterates other, more preferred stories of family pride. While we are drawn to the narrative therapies' emphases on strengths, resources, and the ascendance of positive narratives, we believe that when working with families in which there has been sexual abuse, a premature or exclusive focus on highlighting positive "stories" can obscure the painful realities of the abuse story and the dangers that may still exist. Instead, we assist families to examine both their positive shared experiences and their negative experiences of abuse and betrayal, side by side, without simply substituting the positive for the negative. Both stories now have a place in the history of the child and the family, and the inherent contradictions between the positive and negative experiences with family members cannot easily be eliminated. This is the essence of a "both–and" way of thinking, described shortly.

For example, in one family in which the parents minimized the impact of the abuse of one sibling by another, the therapist asked the parents to describe the things they were proud of in their parenting over the years. After a full, detailed description that included trips they took as a family, cultural events to which they exposed the children, and how they encouraged academic achievement, the therapist asked them if they were proud of their dedication and love for their children. Once the parents knew that the therapist saw them positively, they more easily faced the painful, traumatic effects of the abuse on themselves and their children.

Multiple Perspectives

Each family member—and other persons involved with the family—holds a particular perspective on any particular event or aspect of their lives, and no one perspective is inherently "better" than any other. Descriptions of a family's "reality" that highlight the similarities *and* differences among perspectives (and the resulting tensions) often capture the family's experience more closely than do attempts to find the "main" or overall "truth." Professionals, too, only hold a perspective, which is not inherently better than those of families, although the societally sanctioned power of professionals to diagnose and describe often prioritizes their perspectives over those of families.

We reflect this both–and stance in the way we speak with families. Even when we disagree strongly with a position taken by members of the family, we will preface our statement with something like "based on our experience." For example, in one family, a mother believed the 10-year-old daughter was at fault for the abuse because she had not listened to the mother's admonishments not to tease her 15-year-old stepbrother. The therapist asked the mother to describe the teasing, her beliefs about gender and entitlement to sex, her sense of what other family members felt about the daughter's culpability, as well as her sense of the stepbrother's general character and personal history. After inviting and carefully listening to the mother's full elaboration of her views, the therapist said that in her experience, working with abuse and families, it seemed easier sometimes for family members to blame the abused girl for the son's abusive behavior than to hold him accountable. She spoke of other families with whom she had worked, in which girls tease but the brothers had not responded by sexually molesting them. In other words, without devaluing the mother's views, the therapist offered her a different perspective. The mother listened intently and nondefensively, and then spontaneously speculated about why the stepson behaved as he did. Her new explanation did not blame the victimized daughter. As we discuss later in this chapter, our general belief in the need to hear all perspectives of all family members does not mean we automatically give all perspectives equal standing or credence. Rather, we privilege the perspectives conducive to creating safety for the child and nonoffending family members.

"Both–And" versus "Either–Or" Thinking

Seemingly contradictory thoughts, perceptions, and feelings—and the dynamic tension experienced in holding two or more seemingly discrepant views—can characterize a person's or family's sense of what is "true" about themselves and their lived experience. In this view, personal and group identity is a complex fabric made up of many "strands" of meaning—each strand representing another aspect of the overall life narrative. Each strand or aspect may vary from the next in terms of the persons and contexts involved, the time frame, the roles played by each person, feelings experienced, and so on. Thus, a person has many self-accounts. This notion of a flexible, fluid self shaped by social context and community is in contrast to the traditional notion of an "essential" self that remains the same across all situations (Gergen, 1991). The notion of both–and thinking is to hold the tension of these often contradictory feelings so that one does not have to deny one set of feelings in order to have a coherent life narrative. The "both–and" approach invites people to describe themselves in a manner that includes the entire spectrum of their feelings, thoughts, and behavior in all their complexity. The notion of multiple perspectives and of substituting "both–and" for "either–or" thinking is at the core of our practice of assisting family members to bring forward all of their seemingly contradictory experiences, and of recognizing the inherent emotional complexity of the incest experience.

For example, a mother whose husband abused her child (he was the child's stepfather) for 6 months expressed feelings of outrage, betrayal, and confusion about how she could love someone capable of carrying out such abuse. The therapist encouraged her to elaborate these feelings and empathized with the relational trauma that followed her daughter's disclosure.

After a lengthy exchange on these feelings, the therapist asked about other experiences she had with her husband, ones in which he acted consistent with how she generally viewed him. Once these alternate positive descriptions were brought forth, the mother said quietly, "I guess he is both good and bad." Through this both–and description, she could hold wildly contradictory beliefs and feelings about her husband, and it led to dramatically less confusion and self-blame.

At the broadest level, the impact of social constructionism on our work has been to provide a set of ideas and practices that assist us in considering how the family as a whole, as well as each individual family member, constructs both their collective and individual *identities*, how problems can come to dominate these identities, how families can recover and build upon their preferred self-descriptions, and how new action and new experience strengthen each other in this process of redefining both the collective and individual senses of self. Given the actual and potential impact of sexual abuse on the child's emerging sense of self, and the relationship between family self-definition and the child's self-definition, social constructionist ideas and practices have been quite useful in our work of assisting children and families to recover their identities following the often overwhelming impact of sexual abuse.

IDEAS AND PRACTICES FROM FEMINISM

For the feminist family therapist, the clinical hour must respond to the often perilous status of women and children. The therapist must be prepared to take a stand, to advocate, and to challenge stereotypical expectations surrounding gender that result in the unequal rights and privileges accorded to men and women. Feminist family therapists believe that many interactions are shaped by the basic inequality of the gender arrangements between men and women in our culture. Therefore, these therapists tease out and challenge the gender assumptions that drive a family's cycle of interaction (Sheinberg, 1992). Feminism highlights the need to enlarge the influence of fairness, justice, and equality as core values in family relations (Hare-Mustin & Marecek, 1994).

James and MacKinnon (1990) summarize well the feminist position on sexual abuse:

> The feminist account of incest takes, as its point of departure, the emotional havoc experienced by women and child victims of incest who are

powerless in relation to the offender. Fathers are viewed as having power greater than that of the other family members, reflecting the status of men within the wider socio-economic system. Incest results from the father's abuse of this power. The structure of a patriarchal nuclear family is seen as intrinsic to the problem of incest in two ways: (a) patriarchy enshrines men's dominance over women and children, thus creating the conditions for incest to occur; (b) and the patriarchal nuclear family nurtures the reproduction of gender, i.e., masculinity and femininity. (p. 73, references excluded)

We have observed that even men who do not fit this stereotypical image of a patriarchal, dominant figure—in fact, who may even appear mild and unassertive—still seem to hold basic assumptions about their entitlement to act on their sexual needs and impulses. In our work, we draw on four key ideas deriving from feminist theory, both in general and as applied to the areas of sexual abuse and other forms of intimate violence:

1. The impact of gender beliefs on experience and relational behavior
2. The notion of incest as facilitated by a failure of empathy
3. Women as caretakers of men and boys
4. Offending persons taking complete responsibility for the abuse

Impact of Gender Beliefs on Experience and Relational Behavior

In addition to its focus on asserting equal rights for women and dismantling the patriarchal power structure, feminism has highlighted the ways in which our beliefs about each gender, and the differences between them, lead us to construct the social world in particular ways. For instance, in a society in which the defining characteristics of masculinity include aggressiveness, competitiveness, and independence, men are expected, by others and themselves, to get what they seek, not to back down from conflict, and not to experience or show feelings associated with vulnerability—feelings such as hurt, worry, sadness, and the need for care. In addition, if the defining characteristics of femininity are empathy, caretaking, willingness to compromise, dependence upon others, and experiencing and expressing feelings associated with vulnerability, men come to define themselves as *not female*; therefore, they are not empathic, not dependent, not caretaking, and so on.

From a feminist perspective, then, beliefs about the defining characteristics of men and women—in conjunction with the actual fundamental

power inequity between them—set the stage for abuse and violence perpetrated by men on women and children (Brickman, 1984; Herman, 1981,
1992; James & MacKinnon, 1990). The feminist argument is not that stereotypical beliefs about men and women *cause* men to abuse women. There
are many mediating factors between the presence of gender beliefs and violent, abusive behavior. The feminist point is that these beliefs *facilitate* such
behavior and that change in these basic beliefs—on a personal, case-by-
case basis, as well as on the societal level—could reduce the likelihood of
such behavior.

Feminists point out that stereotypical divisions between men and
women not only present dangers to women, but also present tremendous
limitations on men. Men who rigidly adhere to stereotypical definitions of
what it means to be a man may not allow themselves to experience or acknowledge painful emotions, or to depend upon others during times of
stress. They may also reject empathic feelings and desires to take care of
others, because these impulses do not fit their image of what it is to be a
man. In our work with males who offend, we create the context for examining and reconsidering rigid stereotypes, and for experimenting with new,
more flexible images of manhood.

With one teenage boy who abused his younger sister, although his father berated him on the one hand for the abuse, he supported his son's
objectifying view of women. For instance, he took pleasure and pride in his
attractive son making a game out of seeing how many young women he
could seduce. Through therapy, this young man became more comfortable
with experiencing and expressing feelings of vulnerability (fear, need for
nurturance, insecurity), resulting in a dramatic change in his definition of
masculinity and his view of women.

Incest Facilitated by a Failure of Empathy

One feminist-based hypothesis useful in working with men who offended is
that their abuse of the child was facilitated by a failure of empathy—that
because they do not allow themselves to feel vulnerable, or to relate affec-
tionately to others, they did not imagine the impact of their behavior upon
the child. This idea is echoed by a number of other researchers working in
the field of abuse (see, e.g., Herman, 1981; Parker & Parker, 1986).

However, in our experience working with men who offended the issue
is often not as simple as an inability to empathically imagine the child's experience. Some who offended appear fully able to imagine the feelings of
others, including their victims, and even describe having noticed, during

the abusive act, verbal or nonverbal cues from the victims of the fear, embarrassment, anger, or pain they seemed to experience. Rather, the issue may better be cast in some cases as the offending family member's failure to link empathic perception, feeling, and action. In these cases, the offending family member appears to override any empathic inkling in the service of fulfilling his own needs. Again, in our work, we unpack and bring forward the premises of the offending family member that guide him in these moments of choice.

Women as Caretakers of Men and Boys

Women we work with sometimes hold the perspective that women are responsible for taking care of men, and that men's pride, honor, and self-respect must be safeguarded at all costs—even if it means a woman's (including a girl's) pride, honor, and self-respect must be sacrificed. One part of this belief that many women explicitly or implicitly hold is that women and girls are stronger emotionally than men and boys. To the extent that women view their daughters as extensions of themselves, and since they themselves have put up with criticisms and being excluded by men from various activities, they may assume that this is part of the "reality" of being a woman, *and* that their daughters will be able to cope as they have (see similar points made by Chodorow, 1978). Importantly, from a feminist perspective, these mothers' gender-reifying behavior toward their children—which, when viewed in isolation, might suggest that mothers do much to set the stage for acceptance of abuse—must be viewed within the broader patriarchal context in which women are made to be the "second sex" across generations (de Beauvoir, 1974).

For instance, in one family in which there was sibling incest, the parents were reluctant to engage in therapy. Behind this reluctance was their belief that their daughter would eventually forget about the abuse, but if the boy was subjected to therapy in which he had to speak about what he had done, he might have difficulty functioning in the future as a heterosexual man.

Offending Family Members Must Take Complete Responsibility for the Abuse

One issue central to a feminist perspective on family violence is that of attributing moral responsibility to the offending family member. This issue has shaped positions regarding whether or not to provide treatment to offending persons. As Brickman (1984) has pointed out in her review, some feminists in the area of family violence hold that offending persons "should be punished and not treated. Others believe in treatment, but not as an alternative to criminal action. These apparently harsh views grow from the need to establish crimes within the family as equal in seriousness to the same offenses committed on the public street" (p. 64). Our opinion is that from a consistent feminist perspective that prioritizes the safety and recovery of the child and nonoffending family members (Brickman, 1984), treatment of the offending family member is critical to ensuring that he does not reabuse the child or commit sexual offenses against others. The question of when or whether to include the offending member in *family* treatment, or to support reuniting the offending member with the family, is a separate issue, to be discussed in an upcoming chapter.

Whether or not he is legally prosecuted, from a feminist perspective, the offending family member must always take 100% responsibility for the abuse. Whatever understanding we might construct of the family dynamics that facilitated abuse, including systemic, circular explanations of interactional patterns to which more than one family member contributes and for which more than one member holds responsibility, acts of violence, intimidation, and abuse must be understood from a "linear" perspective in which one person exerts power over the other(s) and holds complete responsibility for these actions (see Goldner, 1998, 1999, and Goldner et al., 1990, for an explication of these ideas as they relate to domestic violence). Holding this clear moral stance regarding the offending member's responsibility for acts of abuse enables us to entertain psychological and systemic explanations regarding the conditions that led up to his *decision* (whether articulated as such to himself or not) to act abusively.

For example, in one family, the husband complained about his peripheral role in the family. His explanation for a drunken episode during which he fondled his stepdaughter (which he claimed not to remember clearly because he had been intoxicated) attributed blame to his wife and stepdaughter for marginalizing him. Although we said we were interested in addressing his dissatisfaction with his perceived place in the family, we could attend to it only after he clearly took responsibility for abusing his stepdaughter. In other words, no matter how he felt, it was his choice to respond to these feelings by abusing her and, therefore, entirely his responsibility.

IDEAS FROM SYSTEMS THERAPIES

Over the past 15 years or so, systems theory as applied to families and family therapy has undergone a shift from reliance on mechanistic, cybernetic, and structural metaphors (and accompanying notions of homeostasis, circular causality, feedback loops, subsystems, boundaries, enmeshment–disengagement, and the like) to reliance on linguistic metaphors and notions about processes of meaning making (Hoffman, 1990; Paré, 1995, 1996; Sheinberg & Penn, 1991; Zimmerman & Dickerson, 1994). On the level of intervention, this shift is reflected in the change from a focus on observing and interrupting behavioral sequences to a focus on eliciting, questioning, and facilitating change in family members' perceptions, beliefs, and feelings.

As our discussion of social constructionist ideas and practices reveals, our work reflects this shift, focusing more on meaning and less on sequences and structure. However, we do hold certain assumptions that preceded the advent of social constructionist thinking in family therapy and can be rightfully attributed to the systems therapies as a group. In particular, we use the following three concepts:

1. The importance of social context in the life of problems
2. The influence of loyalties and attachments
3. The importance of the dimensions of power and closeness

The Importance of Social Context in the Life of Problems

All systems therapies (and social constructionist therapies, for that matter) agree that the problems of individuals occur in social context, which may play a role in sustaining problems or ameliorating them. We consider the impact of multiple levels of context in our work with families and sexual abuse. We work with families to identify which aspects of context create more stress and interfere with healing from the incest, and which serve as actual or potential resources to facilitate this healing. We attend particularly to interfaces between the family and the "larger systems" institutions that get involved following disclosure, and work to facilitate a useful relationship between ourselves, other professionals, and the family.

We are also particularly attuned to the impact of social class, culture, race, religion, and sexual preference on family members' experiences in general; to how they "construct" their families (in terms of membership, activities, internal norms); to determining the degree to which they experience social and economic oppression; and whether they are likely to have encounters with larger systems institutions. In particular, poorer families (which in inner-city areas usually overlap with racial and ethnic minorities, especially blacks and Latinos/Latinas) are more likely to experience secondary trauma than are higher-income families (who are more likely in urban areas to be white), because for poor families, disclosure more often leads to involvement of social service and other social control institutions.

We address class, race, and culture on a case-by-case basis and ask questions that bring forth from each family member the particular meanings these aspects of personhood contribute to his or her experience of the abuse. To illustrate the wide range of meanings that cultural background can contribute to the experience of abuse, consider the following four examples. In one family we saw, the mother of a sexually abused young girl said she grew up believing that women and girls must expect and endure abuse of one sort or another. In her tone and facial expression, she conveyed that she felt resigned to this reality. In contrast, another woman said that there was a belief in her culture that women are responsible for ensuring that children are not abused. Another mother described feeling enormous rage toward her boyfriend, who abused her children. Her rage was intensified because in her culture and religion, women are usually protected by and trusting of men. Still another mother expressed that the public aspect of the disclosure mortified her. In her culture, it is expected that problems are to be handled entirely within the family. The idea of involving outsiders in family affairs upset her more than the abusive incident itself.

Bringing forth the meaning of the abuse and its disclosure ensures that we address first the aspects of experience most relevant to the family being treated. Again, although we assume that there are some similar responses shared by all families that have had this experience, the idiosyncratic meaning for any individual or family is important for us to understand so as to be most helpful (see Fraenkel, 1995, for a discussion of the role of addressing both general and family-specific experiences in family therapy). Similarly, we do not assume that two or more families sharing the same racial, ethnic, class, or religious aspects experience themselves in terms of these aspects in the same way. Like some others (Falicov, 1995), we recognize that each family (and family members within a family) represents a somewhat unique intersection of demographic categories and group memberships, and may identify with and experience their skin color, cultural background, country of origin, religion, or class differently from others in the same groups, and their identifications may change over time.

Another, somewhat thornier aspect of discussing issues of race, class, and culture centers on how to address differences between the therapist and the family. In one family, for instance, we noticed that the mother was quite deferential toward the therapist. When the therapist made a suggestion of any sort, the woman would immediately say how good it was and how she was pleased to learn. As therapy was not mandated, and because there was no legal issue that might have pressured the woman to be extremely cooperative, we wondered if she was responding to the difference between her own and the therapist's race, cultural background, educational level, and class. The therapist raised the possibility, saying that she was thinking about their different backgrounds, and wondered if the woman was also aware of these differences. The woman said she was very much aware of the differences, so the therapist pursued a conversation that led the woman to describe her belief that children from the therapist's race were more successful. She further explained that she wanted to learn about how it was done. The therapist responded to her assumption on two levels. One level was that of ideas, by exploring the woman's definition of success, including the ways in which she felt her cultural practices produced children that were successful in certain ways but not in other ways. The other level was personal. The therapist disclosed some of her trials and tribulations in raising a child, as well as her own ambivalence over some ideas in her culture about child rearing. The discussion was lively, real, and surprising for both women as they articulated the assumptions each brought to the act of parenting. In turn, the discussion led to a much less hierarchical relationship between the therapist and the woman, one in which the woman felt freer to offer her own ideas and solutions, and to evaluate the usefulness of the therapist's suggestions rather than automatically adopting them.

The Influence of Loyalties and Attachments

Therapists and theorists working within the intergenerational tradition (Boszormenyi-Nagy & Spark, 1973; Kerr & Bowen, 1988) have long noted the importance of understanding the impact of loyalties, and mixed loyalties, on the quality of the relationships among family members. When a family member experiences him- or herself as torn between allegiance to two or more family members, conflict can ensue, especially if the person in the loyalty bind feels pressed to align him- or herself more with one person than with another.

One useful concept in understanding the emotional power of family loyalties that has only recently been introduced into the field of family therapy is "attachment," drawn from psychoanalytic and developmental psychology (Byng-Hall, 1995). Originally conceived as a dyadic process between a mother and child or between romantic partners, those working from a systems perspective have noted the impact of the entire family, as well as the family's broader social support network, on the quality of dyadic attachments (Belsky, Rovine, & Fish, 1989; Donley, 1993; see also the review by Byng-Hall, 1995). And just as a secure attachment between a mother and child enables the child comfortably to explore her or his environment, the notion of a secure *family base* is "a family that provides a reliable network of attachment relationships in which all family members of whatever age are able to feel sufficiently secure to explore" (Byng-Hall, 1995, p. 46). Disruptions in one set of relationships—for instance, in the relationship between parents—can affect the security of other attachment relationships, for instance, between the child and her or his parents (Belsky et al., 1989).

When one person acts so as to violate the family's sense of internal security, it can disrupt all of the attachments among family members (Byng-Hall, 1995). Sexual abuse, particularly by the adult male father and partner, can have just such an impact.

From the perspective of a family systems approach that emphasizes issues of attachment, "the role of the therapist is to help to resolve conflicts that threaten relationships, and to explore relevant belief systems that may be contributing to a sense of insecurity" (Byng-Hall, 1995, p. 45). Our work with families in which sexual abuse has occurred centers largely on clarifying loyalties and strengthening safe attachment relationships, and assisting families to create a sense of a secure base, both for the children and the nonoffending adults.

The Importance of the Dimensions of Power and Closeness

Although "traditional" family systems therapies have been justly criticized for proclaiming the universal "healthy" norms regarding patterns of closeness and hierarchy in families, regardless of differences in culture (see Fraenkel, 1997, for a review), we regard the basic dimensions of closeness/connectedness and power/hierarchy as useful for thinking about the nature of problems and strengths in family relationships; that is, problems in families generally center on issues of who's close to whom or distant from whom in what particular ways and settings, and around issues of how power and influence are distributed among family members. We are interested in family members' *perceptions, beliefs, and desires* regarding the patterns of closeness/connectedness and power/hierarchy in their relationships and draw no assumptions about the nature of their relationships from observing their behavior without first understanding family members' points of view.

In summary, our conception of systemic thinking centers on how families within and across generations construct meanings, and how these meanings inform family interaction and constrain families' flexibility and capacity for change. This conception of systemic thinking is different from one that centers on observing and attempting directly to alter—through strategic language and tasks—repetitive, unproductive behavioral sequences among family members. When we conceptualize systems-oriented work as centered around processes of family meaning making, contradictions between social constructionist and systems approaches fade, and convergences appear.

Although our major focus is on experienced meaning, we also engage with families to assist them to change patterns of action. Like others influenced by social constructionist ideas (White & Epston, 1990), we recognize the power of action patterns to sustain nonpreferred meanings, and the power of change in behavior to elicit and establish new meaning. In addition, families—particularly those struggling with a crisis such as sexual abuse—often need assistance with such action-oriented issues as safety planning, changing communication styles (e.g., finding ways to talk about problems without escalations), and helping children with concrete behavioral difficulties. In most cases, family members describe to us these problematic patterns. However, if we observe a pattern that seems potentially problematic, which the family has not mentioned, we share our observations with the family in a manner that invites discussion about the pattern's meaning and the family's preferences regarding it, rather than intervening through directives or reframes.

INTEGRATING SOCIAL CONSTRUCTIONIST, FEMINIST, AND SYSTEMS THINKING

In fact, there are common themes among these three perspectives as well as some important differences. The key differences among the three approaches center on conceptions of power, the nature of reality, therapist expertise, and the relationship between meaning and action.

Feminist Critiques of Systems and Social Constructionist Theories: A Focus on Power

Feminists have critiqued systems conceptualizations of violence and sexual abuse (and of other problems, for that matter) that view the abuse as a homeostatic mechanism that serves to stabilize a family threatened by the potential dissolution of a key family relationship (i.e., the parents' marriage) or by the incipient departure of one or more family members (Carter, Papp, Silverstein, & Walters, 1986; James & MacKinnon, 1990; Libow, Raskin, & Caust, 1982; see Alexander, 1985, and the review by James & MacKinnon, 1990, for traditional systems explanations of incest). More broadly, conceptualizations of incest as being an outgrowth of a "dysfunctional" family system (Trepper & Barrett, 1989; Trepper & Neidner, 1996) are rejected by feminists. Rather than being a symptom that holds a family together or a problem particular to families with dysfunctional organization, abuse is viewed from a feminist perspective as symptomatic of the gender-based power differences that simultaneously threaten the safety of women and children—providing them with a good reason for leaving an abusive man—and keep them trapped because of their financial and material dependence on the more powerful man (James & MacKinnon, 1990). As James and MacKinnon (1990) write, "By viewing incest as a phenomenon particular to the interactional patterns of dysfunctional families, feminists argue that therapists obscure the nature of power relationships between males and females, both within the family and between the family and wider society" (p. 71).

From a feminist position, lack of recognition of the fundamental power differences between men and women in families also led some systems-oriented therapists to develop notions of incest as due primarily to female partners/mothers being unresponsive to the sexual and emotional needs of their male partners—the quality or quantity of which are not questioned in these formulations—and to the security needs of their daughters. This latter formulation implies that the mother is responsible for protecting the daughter from the father's abuse rather than the father (or other male family member) being responsible for modulating his own sexual impulses and behavior. In some systems formulations, the mother's deficits as partner and parent have been linked intergenerationally to her family-of-origin experiences, including a history of being abused herself as a child. Rather than focusing on the unique dynamics of the mother's family of origin that resulted in personal deficits, the feminist therapist would more likely hypothesize that the mother grew up in a patriarchal family in which she was taught that she could not, and should not, protect herself and that this belief may have informed her choice of a partner and her fear of stopping his abusive behavior.

Application of systems thinking has also led to a notion of "incest families" as more isolated, and as having rigid "boundaries" around them while having diffuse boundaries among members, leading to incest (Alexander,

1985; Mrazek & Bentovim, 1981; Trepper & Barrett, 1989; see also a recent review by Trepper & Niedner, 1996). Again, in these formulations, there is no attribution of responsibility to a particular family member for such boundary issues. In contrast, from a feminist perspective, when such boundary issues occur, they are generally viewed as the result of constraints imposed by a dominating male figure, often *after* abuse has begun (James & MacKinnon, 1990).

Feminists have also critiqued some of the postmodern notions underlying social constructionist thought and therapeutic practice as potentially dissolving the real, oppressive conditions of many women's lives. For instance, the postmodern rejection of "grand narratives"—beliefs and other explanatory frames meant to describe (and prescribe) certain "truths" for all (or at least, large numbers of) people—serves feminist objectives when it rejects descriptions that prioritize men and disempower women, but it threatens the feminist position when it rejects the possibility of all grand narratives, including that of justice and equality (Hare-Mustin & Marecek, 1994; McNay, 1992). Similarly, some feminists have raised concerns about the postmodern notion that there is no "objective truth," that all is a matter of perspective. Again, this position threatens to delegitimize the feminist view of violence and abuse, and other misuses of power, as real acts with real consequences. As Hare-Mustin and Marecek (1994) have noted, "Feminists have criticized postmodernism's seemingly endless fascination with words and texts to the exclusion of material reality," posing the "risk that a postmodern psychology ignores women's lived experience by retreating into arcane theory" (p. 15). On the broadest level, when gender is deconstructed and the category of "woman" is eliminated as "real" (Butler, 1990), it becomes more difficult to defend the need for a women's movement (Goldner, 1993).

Reconciling Postmodernist and Feminist Views on Power and Reality

On the other hand, as these authors point out, postmodern and social constructionist thinking has highlighted the power of words to define reality and to dictate action. Thus, from a social constructionist point of view, using language to recast sex between fathers and daughters from being assumed as an unspoken right (James & MacKinnon, 1990) to being described as an "abuse" paved the way for programs of action to protect children. If social constructionism is to be consistent with its rejection of the possibility of grand narratives and universal truths, it cannot support the notion that some truths (e.g., the need for equality and justice, the importance of narrative, the fluidity of identity) are more true than others (Held, 1995). On the other hand, its emphasis on the need to recognize multiple perspectives and to give all persons a voice essentially represents another grand narrative (Hare-Mustin & Marecek, 1994), one that we believe embodies the values of fairness and equality.

One of the core ideas of postmodernism is that all knowing, observing, and acting—including that of social scientists and other experts—are situated in historical traditions and values, bound by language, and, therefore, cannot directly access "objective reality" (Gergen, 1985; McNamee & Gergen, 1992). This idea has sometimes been wrongly critiqued as suggesting that because an "objective reality" is deemed unknowable, any belief is as good as the next one (Held, 1995), or that constructionists cannot hold beliefs.

Rather, we and others (Efran & Clarfield, 1992) view a consistent social constructionist stance as maintaining that we cannot *avoid* having beliefs, and that professionals need to articulate theirs (to colleagues as well as clients) and the bases for holding them. To acknowledge that others may construct the world differently and that there is no objective basis for choosing one value system over another does not mean that we cannot, or should not, hold and attempt to promote certain values. In this view, what is deemed "true" and "right" is established through dialogue and through building communities: In Efran and Clarfield's words, " 'truth' is a set of opinions widely shared" (1992, p. 201).

This belief in the community basis of "truth," and in the importance of language in constructing meaning and action, affects our work not only with individual families but also with larger systems. It has fueled our efforts to build a consortium of agencies in New York that now work in coordinated fashion with families in which sexual abuse has occurred (Peck et al., 1995). Our training programs, both within the consortium, in our broader community of New York City, and elsewhere, are meant to provide a common language and approach to sexual abuse that will enable better communication among professionals and, therefore, more consistent treatment for families.

Following from the point about therapists' need to be explicit about beliefs, in our work with sexually abused children and their families, we have chosen to prioritize feminist beliefs that highlight the manner in which power is often misused within societies, and families, by men; that the oppression by men of women and children is real and not an epistemological error; and that this societal and familial subtext facilitates, but does not cause, sexual abuse. Our choice of a feminist "frame" as our foundational belief is based on our belief in equality, fairness, and justice. As we noted earlier, this foundational belief gives us a clear moral perspective regarding who is responsible for the abuse.

However, our use of systems and social constructionist perspectives also emerges from our basic values. We view families as working best when all members' needs and perspectives are heard and included, and believe that a core role of parents is both to model these values for children and to exemplify them in the decisions they make. Thus, we find all three perspectives consistent with the values of equality, fairness, and justice.

An Integrative Notion of Therapist Expertise

In addition to different ideas about power in society and in families, traditional systems, feminist, and social constructionist perspectives also differ in beliefs about the *therapist's* use of power. Traditional systems approaches have been critiqued by both the social constructionist and feminist perspectives as relying on the therapist's assumption of expertise greater than that of families themselves, and the use of this expert role to direct change in the family (Fraenkel, 1997; Libow, Raskin, & Caust, 1982; McNamee & Gergen, 1992). Systems therapists have been critiqued for the belief that they can observe and deduce the meaning of family patterns without asking family members how they understand these patterns, and without recognizing their involvement in the observed system (Hoffman, 1985, 1990).

However, in our view, this construction of the therapist role is particular to certain schools of systems therapy and is not a necessary condition of systems-oriented thinking and therapy in general, the essence of which is understanding family problems in context. In our integration, we have adopted the feminist and social constructionist emphasis on collaboration with families. Like others, we strongly believe that the "transformations" sought in therapy or in work with larger social systems "cannot be undertaken by a single will, an all-knowing or all-seeing expert. Rather, transformation is inherently a relational matter, emerging from myriad coordinations among persons" (McNamee & Gergen, 1992, p. 5).

At the same time, like other feminist (Libow et al., 1982) and social constructionist therapists (Efran & Clarfield, 1992), we recognize the unavoidable and potentially useful hierarchy between therapists and clients, and the need to handle this power responsibly (Efran & Clarfield, 1992)—a point first made explicit long ago by such "traditional" systems thinkers as Jay Haley (1963). We do view ourselves as "evolving experts" in helping families solve their problems and in the area of sexual abuse, but we use our accumulated experience only as a starting point. We approach each new family as unique in its particular history, situation, experiences, ways of interpreting events, and constellation of problems and strengths, and also recognize ways in which family members may suffer from certain experiences common to many children and families in which there has been sexual abuse.

Reconciling Feminism and Social Constructionism with a Systems Perspective: Emphasis on Relational Meaning versus Behavioral Observation

Both feminist and social constructionist thinkers also critique traditional family systems therapies for the application of mechanistic notions such as homeostasis, feedback loops, and the like—feminists, because these notions obscure male responsibility for misuse of power, and social constructionists, largely because they obscure the unique story of each family within a general theory appropriated from the study of nonhuman phenomena (Paré, 1995). Embedded in the social constructionist critique is also the belief that therapy is about exploring families' processes of meaning making, not about observing and altering patterns of behavior.

As we have noted, our view of systems therapy centers on these processes of family meaning making. However, we also hold that there is value in working directly with families to change unsatisfying patterns of action that may serve to sustain particular meanings. We do so without any recourse to notions of homeostasis or feedback loops—only to the notion that certain patterns become habitual and affect how family members see each other and themselves, which in turn leads to more of the same behavior. In this sense, action patterns are relational beliefs in motion.

We agree with McNamee and Gergen (1992) when they write that "our conjoint formulations of what is the case are typically embedded within our patterns of action" (p. 5). However, while they make this statement to support a focus on the "formulations," we suggest that the statement argues equally for a focus on action. Sometimes, change begins at the level of meaning, providing direction for change at the level of action. Likewise, change sometimes needs to proceed at the level of action before meanings can shift: Families may need to try something new, adopting an attitude of experimentation and creativity in the face of the unknown, and see how this affects their feelings and beliefs. Often, changes begin at each level simultaneously and mutually inform each other.

In summary, our integration of systems, feminist, and social constructionist perspectives, which we call the "relational" approach, achieves the following:

- Views clarifying all relationships, and strengthening positive relationships, as the core of therapy
- Centers on how families make sense of their relational experiences and on changing beliefs that create problems and restrict possibilities
- Examines all problems in multiple contextual layers
- Is based on promoting the values of equality, fairness, and justice in families
- Prioritizes feminist-based concerns about misuse of power in families and in the broader society
- Eschews mechanistic systems ideas but retains the notion that patterns of interaction can encapsulate and restrict meaning and are worthy targets of intervention
- Includes intervention levels of both meaning and action, often simultaneously

The Value of Theoretical Eclecticism: Therapeutic Checks and Balances

The previous discussion of differences and convergence among the three primary theoretical perspectives that contribute to the relational approach demonstrates how a multitheoretical approach enriches thinking about as complex a phenomenon as incest. In actual work with a particular family, the three perspectives provide checks and balances in our thinking about a family. This is illustrated in case examples throughout the book.

PART II

Implementing the Relational Approach

Chapter Four

Incest as a Complex Story

I n this chapter, we focus on the ideas and practices we use to assist families to recognize and manage one of the most painful and confusing of all the effects of incest: the manner in which the act of abusing a child in the family contorts and complicates all the relationships in the family. The child and nonoffending family members often feel they do not know how to think or feel about themselves, each other, the member who offended, and the family as a whole. Unfortunately, but understandably, one of the most common reactions of families, and sometimes of the professionals working with them postdisclosure, is to attempt to cope with the relational trauma by reducing complexity through creating a simpler "story" about the abuse and everyone's feelings. As we discuss, this effort is ultimately ineffective, as it does not honor the inherent relational complexity that incest creates. We offer here ideas and approaches to helping families comes to terms with this complexity.

NARRATIVES AND IDENTITY: STORIES OF PRIDE AND SHAME

Basic Concepts

In our work, we think about the incest experience as the family's "story of shame." It is only among a number of other stories, others of which are

75

positive, that the family can recount and tell about itself. We work to elicit conversations among family members about these positive stories, which we call "stories of pride," and help them build upon these pride stories even as they contend with the effects of the abuse story. The goal is for family members eventually to experience the possibility of having multiple, coexisting narratives and not push out the story of shame and replace it with positive narratives, but instead, to be able to view themselves as a family that lived the story of abuse while at the same time living and continuing to live other, more positive stories of pride.

Guidelines for Practice

The first and most important step in translating these ideas into practice is that the therapist's attitude as a professional working with the child and her family must reflect a basic respect for them as people, struggling to come to terms with a shameful, potentially stigmatizing experience. One way to show this attitude is to ask about and take interest in the family's strengths and resourcefulness from the very beginning, both in dealing with the abuse and in general. In early contacts, the therapist sympathizes with the difficulties they have experienced during the period of the abuse and following disclosure, asks about how they handled these difficulties, and recognizes the ways in which they showed resourcefulness in dealing with these challenging experiences both individually and as a family. In addition, the therapist lets family members know that he or she is interested in them as people apart from their problems, and does not view them as defined solely by their problems, by asking each of them as soon as the opportunity arises about positive aspects of their work (including asking children about their school life), their interests, hobbies, family activities, and so on, that is, areas of their lives about which they experience pride and a sense of competency.

Often when families first make contact with the system of professionals, the aftermath of the abuse and disclosure may preoccupy them, and they may have difficulty talking about anything else for a time. In addition, when families are mandated to therapy, the adults in particular may believe that they are "here to talk about the abuse" and need to show the therapist that they will be cooperative clients and responsible parents by focusing solely on the abuse. The therapist can encourage and legitimize discussion of other topics by saying something like, "You've told me quite a bit about the abuse and how it has affected everyone. I'd be interested to know more about the things that make you feel proud—each of you individually and as a family."

As the therapist shows interest and supports the expansion of the family's strengths and sources of pride—even as he or she explores with family members the shameful story of the abuse—and assists them to use their resources to overcome the effects of the abuse, family members come to see that both stories can coexist and the story of shame eventually ceases to define them. The use of "both–and" thinking illustrated later in this chapter, also greatly assists in freeing family members to consider themselves in more complex ways.

One more specific practice we developed to elicit prideful aspects between a mother and child is called the similarities/differences/pride exercise. We only use this exercise when there appear to be strained or outright negative feelings between mother and child (which we, like others [Joyce, 1997], find not always or even mostly the case), as it is excellent for strengthening the parent–child bond. Meeting with parent and child, we first ask the parent to describe some of the ways in which she perceives herself and her child to be *similar* to each other; then, ways she perceives herself and her child to be *different*; and finally, things about her child that make her *proud*.

Second, we ask the child to list ways in which she sees herself as *different* from her parent; then, ways she sees herself as *similar*; and finally, things about her parent that make her *proud*. In general, we try to guide the parent and child to describe mostly positive qualities about themselves and the other, although when it comes to differences, they may express aspects of each other's (or their own) personality or behavior that they regard as less positive. In particular, sometimes the parent needs gentle encouragement at first to focus on *positive* attributes when listing similarities and sources of pride: It is often easy for the parent who is somewhat angry with her child to drift into talking about problems and negative attributes.

We ask the *parent* to begin with a description of *similarities*, because she is often so ready to talk about the differences (usually in a negative way), and we want immediately to set the tone of a positive experience that will ultimately bring parent and child together. On the other hand, we ask the *child* to begin by listing *differences*, because children, especially adolescents, often feel uncomfortable describing the similarities between themselves and their parents.

We have found that this exercise has several useful outcomes. First, it can help the estranged parent and child relocate and express positive perceptions, feelings, and thoughts about each other. Recognizing positive feelings in themselves about the other, and hearing the other name positive qualities about themselves, can assist parent and child to soften their sense of distance or negative feelings for each other, to begin to heal old hurts resulting from previous insults, and to draw closer together. Second, it identifies potential new or renewed areas for parent–child involvement and identification with each other. As parent and child come to recognize their interests, personal qualities, and abilities, these also can become the basis for a closer connection.

Third, the exercise allows parent and child to begin to discuss in a structured, safe way their differences and the concerns each may have about the other. In one family, the therapist's exploration of a mother's and daughter's sources of pride in each other strengthened their relationship. The relationship had been weakened by an earlier period in which the child was sent away without warning by the mother to live with relatives, and ended up living in a shelter, from where her mother then recovered her. The mother's struggle with the exercise of listing things she was proud of about her daughter (she had difficulty sticking to positives and tended to drift back into problems) led to recognition on her part that she feared complimenting her daughter too much, lest she develop an inflated sense of herself. Exploration of the mother's own childhood revealed that her parents also did not give her feedback about some of her strengths, and that she might have unwittingly been passing along to her daughter a sense that one should not be too confident in oneself, especially as a woman. In the mother's case, her parents had never told her the contents of her grammar and high school report cards, and that she was receiving good grades; she had always assumed she was a C or D student but was in fact getting B's. Only upon receiving her transcript to apply to college did she realize how well she had done in high school; in retrospect, she felt that, had she known, she would have tried harder to be an A student.

Thus, the pride exercise with her daughter not only strengthened the mother–daughter relationship but it also led this woman to reflect upon how her academic and career success had been interfered with first by her parents, then by her husband, and now by her boyfriend (the man who abused her daughter), and strengthened her determination to move and pursue career training, with or without her boyfriend.

Another exercise we use, particularly in sessions with more than two family members, is to have members list on a blackboard things about the family that make them proud. This can be useful in sessions with either the abused child or a juvenile who has offended. Especially in work with families of juveniles who offended, when the family is having difficulty holding the offending child responsible for his actions, encouraging the family to identify sources of pride, including pride in nonabusive behaviors of the juvenile who offended, can help family members lower their denial and fully face his offending behavior. The following example illustrates the power of eliciting stories of pride in work with a juvenile who offended and his family.

Example

In one family, exploration of sources of family pride and continuity allowed a juvenile who offended to feel more comfortable openly discussing what he had done to his younger female cousin, and allowed the other family members to stop minimizing the impact of the abuse on the cousin (who had since moved with her parents to another city). In an early session, Randy, the 11-year-old offending boy, was asked who he thought would be the last person to forgive him if he openly acknowledged abusing his 7-year-old cousin Angela. He said he would be the last, and that he would hate himself. This captured the dilemma for Randy and other family members, namely, that to admit to the abuse and its impact would lead to a sense of overwhelming shame. The therapists in the case saw that in order for Randy to take responsibility for his actions without the acknowledgment destroying him, it would be useful to consider the abuse the "story of shame" and to explore the family's recent and remote history for stories of pride.

The work of restoring stories of pride began when the therapist asked Randy whom he wanted to find out more about in his family. Randy chose his father, Sam. Sam described growing up in California and being raised by his grandmother, facts that Randy had not known. Randy became excited and curious and actively engaged in the process of exploring his father's past. A result of this exploration was Sam's recognition that he had missed having contact with his own father, his sadness at not being closer to Randy, and his resolve to be more involved in Randy's life in the future. The therapist then asked Randy if he would rather talk a bit about "the other story" alone or with his father present. Randy chose to meet with the therapist alone, and for the first time revealed what he had done to Angela, and his feelings of jealousy and anger toward her.

In the next family session, the therapist asked each member to write on the chalkboard something about the family that made him or her feel proud. The mother, Jeanne, expressed pride in her children's successes in school, and in how the family had faced the current crisis together. Other family members also expressed pride about how they had handled the crisis. The therapist then had the family members express a worry, which led the youngest child to share his fear of being "taken away." Other family members shared this fear as well. The conversation then turned back to sources of pride. The father described his pride in the family's ability to be loving and supportive. The therapist then asked who else was proud of the family, and Randy said he was: "They're always there for me. When I need help I can always go to somebody." He listed in particular his mother, whom he also noted always turned out "to be right," even when what she advised him to do often at first seemed "wrong" to him. Naming this support and confidence in the mother's judgment set the stage for a later session in which his mother and father helped Randy to acknowledge to them that he had abused his cousin, and provided him with emotional support and acceptance afterwards.

Randy then went on to list skills and talents of his own in which he took pride. His mother was then asked to list aspects of herself that made her feel proud. She noted how proud she was of her efforts to provide a good role model for her children. Asked if he looked up to his mother, Randy said he did and described how peer pressure to pull pranks often made it difficult to model himself after his mother and follow her requests that he behave himself in school. He reflected that when he misbehaved, he got mad at himself, because he thought he had let his mother down. Turning to the mother, the therapist asked if Randy had ever told her that, and she said, "No, but I sense it." This then became the entry point for discussing further "stories of shame"—first, events not related to the abuse, and later, the abuse itself. Once again, in a subsequent individual meeting, Randy continued to discuss the abuse. It seemed that the prior meeting with his family, sharing sources of pride and worry, lent him the sense of support he needed in order to discuss this difficult, shame-invoking material.

THE PATH OF "BOTH–AND": RECOGNIZING COMPLEX ATTACHMENTS AND IDENTITY

Basic Concepts

The "both–and" framework is a particularly important guide in our work with families in which incest has occurred. As we noted earlier in this chapter, abused children and their families often experience pressure from well-meaning extended family members and from therapists and other professionals to simplify their experiences with incest into a story of good and evil, in which the abused child, siblings, and nonoffending parent are cast as united, vulnerable, and helpless against the offending family member. In this version of the incest drama, child victims should be *only* hurt and angry, and should completely reject the abuser; abusers are *only* evil, bad to their core, and mothers are *only* righteous and indignant. Unfortunately, the idea that this simple story is correct has been reinforced by some of the same media coverage that has raised public consciousness about incest. Many of the families we've seen in therapy have told us that they became extremely confused when they contrasted their complex feelings about the incest experience with the sensational, clichéd, oversimplified story of incest that is sometimes portrayed in the media. Whatever its source, this simplified version of their story distorts family members' experiences and caricatures their feelings, which are usually quite complex and seemingly contradictory.

Often, family members' greatest feelings of shame emanate from the hidden recognition of their continued attachment to the member who offended. The relational approach to therapy encourages members to describe and honor these complex feelings and attachments. By doing so, families can better distinguish safe from unsafe ways of maintaining these attachments. Although it may seem counterintuitive, we have found that the road to family healing from incest is for therapists to bring forth not only feelings of anger and betrayal, but also feelings of love, caring, and loyalty for the abusive man, and to honor these feelings when they exist.

Guidelines for Practice

The foremost guideline in translating the notion of "both–and" possibilities is for the therapist to fight his or her own natural tendency to reduce and simplify people's experiences. Rather, it is important to maintain a flexible, inquiring attitude toward the child and her family as they relate their account of the abuse and their experiences. The therapist needs to look for opportunities to allow the family members to express a variety of feelings, even those that might seem shameful or wrong, such as those that represent their ongoing attachment to the person who offended. Also, the therapist can normalize these complex feelings and the resulting tensions. A good question to ask while listening to family members relate their feelings and experiences is, "Do you have any *other* feelings about or descriptions of (whatever aspect of the abuse the members are talking about—the person who offended, what happened, how they acted in the situation, etc.)?" The emphasis is on helping the child and other family members to consider and express multiple and often contradictory feelings, without feeling obligated to select one over the other (Sheinberg, 1992).

Examples

The following statement by a child reflecting upon the relationship between herself and her abusive father captures the spirit of taking a both–and approach: "I used to feel ashamed that I missed my father. Now, I know I love him and am angry at him. Not at me." Another child, at the end of the session in which she had talked about her anger and love for her abusive father, drew a picture. It was of a smiling girl who she said felt good. Under the picture she wrote, "I love him. I am so angry for what he did to me."

We designed one exercise particularly for young children (ages 4 to 7) to elicit both–and descriptions: the "Thumbs Up Thumbs Down" Game. You introduce the game by asking the child if she can play a game to learn more about the people in her family (this exercise can be done in individual or family sessions). You then ask the child to list all the people in her family and write these names one after the other across the top of the board. Beneath each name are two columns, one labeled with a plus sign (+) and the other with a minus sign (–). You explain that the plus sign is for things the child likes about each family member—"Thumbs up!" The minus sign is for things the child does not like about each family member— "Thumbs down!" You then ask the child to pick a family member to discuss and choose either a Thumbs Up or Thumbs Down "thing" (usually a personal quality, activity, or event done with the child) to say first about that person. If the child names something positive, you next ask her to say something "Thumbs Down" (or vice versa), thereby introducing multiple descriptions of the person. You ask if it is okay to write these things on the board. (In some cases, the child may not want to write certain qualities or events on the board, possibly because this makes them too real again.) In one case, with a particularly physically active child, the therapist became a human board game dial, arm outstretched and finger pointing, spinning around and then back and forth between the positive and negative categories until the child said "Stop!" to select a category.

The exercise is flexible: After stating something about a family member in one category, the child can then go on to state something in the other category, or can pick someone else about whom to talk. Given that the things children at this age describe about others usually refer to events that occur or occurred between them and the other, the game often directly elicits important material about the child's core family relationships that is often difficult to elicit through more direct questions.

Both–and thinking is extremely helpful in working with nonoffending mothers. One of the most complex emotions for a mother at the time of disclosure is when she has strong positive as well as negative feelings toward her abusive partner. Though the negative feelings are acceptable to her, as well as to the world at large, her feelings of love are regarded as wrong and even crazy. Unless the mother is encouraged to articulate her full range of feelings and allowed to honor feelings of attachment to her partner, her support for her child may be problematic. If the therapist does not elicit the mother's positive feelings, those feelings will remain covert and shameful, and she may become socially isolated and less available to her child. Or she may develop ambivalent support—saying the "right" thing but feeling angry with her child for forcing her to choose between child and partner. If mother and therapist coconstruct a nonpathologizing explanation for her attachment to her partner, moral clarity can replace shameful confusion.

The following case example describes a woman whose enduring, secret bond to her partner initially blinded her to her daughter's abuse, and shows how, through recognizing this bond and seeing it as a sign of her compassion, not of her weakness, she was able to revive her sense of self-worth and gain the moral clarity she needed to detach from this man and fully protect her daughter. The therapist helped her by developing the idea that she could hold not only different but also contradictory feelings toward her abusive partner. The vignette also demonstrates how deeply the mother blamed herself for not believing what she knew, and how the therapist helped her develop an explanation of her blinding attachment based on her own history.

Liz came to her first therapy session alone. Her only daughter had told her teacher that her stepfather had abused her for several years. Liz was a thin, attractive woman, who was so nervous that she barely paused between what seemed like disconnected thoughts. However, it was the following statement that most struck the therapist and offered an entry into the key themes in Liz's experience of the abuse: "I am here to speak about a person who harmed us, or that I allowed to do a lot of harm to us. But I can't help but feel sorry for people like that." In this one sentence, Liz captured the dilemma for so many women. She recognized that she had allowed her husband, Harry, to harm the child she loved, and that, despite his abusive behavior, she could not feel what she believed society expected her to feel—total hate for him and no sympathy. Her fast-talking, nervous manner seemed related to her concern that the therapist, too, would blame and condemn her. After all, she acknowledged that she allowed him to harm her child.

The therapist suggested that Liz could be angry with her spouse for what he did and at the same time feel compassion toward him. By describing it in this way, she let Liz know that she, the therapist, accepted that positive as well as negative feelings toward one's partner can coexist even when that partner has been extremely abusive.

In this instance, the simple recognition that it was both possible and acceptable to feel what seemed like mutually exclusive feelings, brought Liz tremendous relief. This insight allowed her to calm down and begin to reflect on why she did, indeed, feel so sorry for Harry. Liz's acceptance of her caring feelings for Harry allowed her to try to answer questions about her motivation for staying with him. These questions, so often buried in a mother's shame about the incest, were crucial to Liz's coming to recognize the forces that could keep Harry in her life and therefore perpetuate the daughter's abuse. It is the answer to these questions about loyalty and emotional bonds that often makes the difference between women who remain and those who leave an abusive relationship unless it changes.

Because Liz was terribly ashamed of her positive feelings for Harry, the therapist had to find a way to explain them that would honor and respect Liz's attachment. As we have seen so often, Liz's positive feelings for Harry came from a part of her that identified with him. Both Harry and Liz had childhoods filled with extraordinary rejection and pain. When Harry confided in Liz, she felt deep empathy, and whenever things went well for her, she wanted to share them with him. When Harry was mean toward her, she believed his explanation that she had done something to cause it. When friends and family tried to get her to leave him, she felt there was a bond with him that they didn't understand and that she couldn't explain—a bond that only she and Harry shared. The secret bond was between the two lost and rejected children. Only after the therapist honored this bond was Liz able to trust her enough to share more and more of her positive feelings for Harry.

In a later meeting, Liz reflected upon that first session. She told the therapist: "The most important thing that you gave me that day is that you spoke about my compassion for this 'lost child' in Harry. That made me feel wonderful, because it gave me a sense of sanity. Other people said that I stayed with him because I have low self-esteem, and that has been very destructive for me. To explain my staying because I am compassionate has allowed me to decide to stay away from him. Now, I feel that there are two people that have to be saved. I can only save one, and it's going to be my daughter. There's no contest."

From our perspective, it was the therapist's comfort with a "both–and" perspective that allowed her to work with Liz to develop an honorable explanation of her attachment to the offending partner rather than driving her feelings underground in order to fit a simplified story of the abuse experience in which the mother either is loyal to her daughter or to the abusive partner, but not to both. Recognition of her continued attachment to the abusive partner allowed Liz the clarity to make the decision to end her relationship with the partner in order to protect her daughter.

As this example illustrates, it is the pairing of two principles of the relational approach to therapy—the notion of acknowledging "both–and" complexity and the need to prioritize the child's safety—that allows family members to sort out their conflicting attachments and loyalties. By distinguishing among the many ways in which family members may *feel* about each other (including the offending member) and what needs to be *done* to ensure that no further abuse occurs, family members can be encouraged to discuss openly their positive feelings about the offending member and at the same time take steps to protect the child against further incidents. In fact, bringing hidden loyalty conflicts out in the open is often a key step to addressing possible blocks in fully protecting the child.

We emphasize here sorting out nonoffending members' mixed feelings about the offending member because, as these examples demonstrate, these feelings are often at the root of other mixed feelings and loyalty conflicts that family members experience toward one another. However, as we have discussed earlier, the "both–and" perspective is useful in assisting family members to address all of their mixed feelings—about each other as well as themselves.

Remember that individual sessions (and group sessions, when available) are often extremely useful in allowing family members a more comfortable first opportunity to discuss their conflicted feelings and loyalties toward one another. Once these are "on the table" and have been validated and normalized by the therapist (or by other group members), therapist and family member can engage in a Decision Dialogue around when and how to express those feelings in family sessions.

SUMMARY

In this chapter, we have discussed practices that assist families in navigating the dilemmas produced by the complex feelings about self and other that arise out of the emotional turmoil of incest. These practices help families and their individual members restore a sense of pride and positive connection, which in turn often is necessary for them to examine more closely the story of shame that is incest. These practices also help family members sort out their often wildly conflicting loyalties in a manner that ensures the safety of the child. In Chapter 5, we address practices that build a collaborative relationship between family members and the therapist, and serve further to empower families to safeguard the child while strengthening family resilience and pride.

Chapter Five

Creating a
Collaborative Therapy

By and large, contemporary systemically oriented therapists share a deep belief in respecting the strengths of families to solve their problems and to promote the best interests of all family members. This "resource perspective" is in contrast to a more traditional psychiatric emphasis on psychopathology—on what's wrong with families, on cataloguing the ways in which they are dysfunctional, and on identifying how they often harm their members (see Walsh, 1998, for an excellent review). Yet despite a general emphasis on the strengths of families, when it comes to families in which incest has occurred, systemically oriented therapists often largely abandon the resource perspective and return to a more pathological view. As we describe in Appendix A, much of the writing and treatment approaches put forward by systems therapists, as well as research on families in which incest has occurred, characterizes the entire family as dysfunctional rather than understanding the negative impact on the family of one member engaging in dysfunctional activity. We have argued strongly for why this is a limiting view of such families, but we certainly understand the impetus for this pathologizing characterization. The extreme gravity, and frankly, the horror, of a child being sexually abused by a family member, often over years, and sometimes in a most intrusive, demeaning fashion, can make it difficult to sustain a belief in families' strengths and re-sources in these cases.

This points to one of the key dilemmas for therapists working with families in which incest has occurred, namely, how to balance ensuring the child's safety within the family, and recognizing that there may be non-protective aspects of family relationships, with continued belief in the ther-apeutic efficacy of engaging family members collaboratively in protecting the abused child.

Our position is that even in the most extreme cases of abuse, the fam-ily can be engaged collaboratively in protecting the child. For some fami-lies, this protection may result in the child and family no longer living together. For other families, it may involve the offending parent or sibling permanently living outside the home or being incarcerated. For yet other families, it may be possible to be reunited with a safety plan. Whatever the family's ultimate living configuration, the family continues to exist in the minds of family members and continues to influence the abused child's thoughts, feelings, and self-accounts.

This chapter describes specific practices of working collaboratively with families. These practices are all variations of using the therapy process to provide opportunities for families to regain control and to make deci-sions in the best interests of the child and other nonoffending family mem-bers. Through collaborating with the therapist to build the therapy, families come to "own" the process of change.

SAFETY FIRST: INITIAL STEPS TO ORGANIZING THE TREATMENT

The first opportunity to empower families comes during the first phone call and first sessions, during which one focus is how to organize the treatment. How the treatment is organized can greatly affect the degree to which the child and other family members feel safe. For instance, a key first decision centers on whom should be invited to a first session, and whom to the next session. In Chapter 8, we present a detailed description of a case in which these decisions were quite complicated and important, so we do not de-scribe this issue here. However, one important general point is that we al-ways have a first (and sometimes second) session with the nonoffending adult members (usually the mother, and sometimes other family members in a position to protect the child) prior to meeting with the child. This meeting serves at least four purposes:

1. To allow the parent to describe the nature, history, and aftermath of the abuse and the events around disclosure, without the chance of retraumatizing the child by having her listen (and possibly hear details of which she was unaware).
2. To orient the parent to the relational approach to treatment; to clarify the distinction between therapy and other professional contacts and services the family may have had following disclosure (such as the forensic interview); to respond to her questions and concerns, unfettered by the presence of the child; and to work out logistics of the appointments.
3. To begin to build a collaborative relationship with the parent (e.g., the adult treatment "subsystem") prior to meeting the child.
4. To get a sense of the degree to which the parent emotionally supports the child and believes her account of the abuse. It is important to work with these issues prior to holding a conjoint session with mother and daughter. Chapter 6 discusses practices for working with parents who are emotionally blocked from supporting their abused children.

Another issue around organizing the treatment includes ensuring that the family now has a viable plan to safeguard the child in the home. If such a plan is not in place, all other topics take a backseat until the therapist is quite sure that the family can protect the child from further abuse. Because it is important as much as possible to separate social control from therapeutic interventions, the issue of establishing and monitoring the child's physical safety in the home is best carried out by another professional, typically someone in CPS, with whom the therapist hopefully has a good working relationship. However, even when CPS has determined that the child is safe, the therapist may ascertain otherwise and need to work with the family, sometimes in conjunction with the CPS worker, to revise the plan.

ONGOING ORGANIZING OF THE TREATMENT: CHOOSING TREATMENT MODALITIES

Although organizational issues highlighted at the onset of treatment (such as whom to invite and when) may continue and provide opportunities for collaborative decision making with families, the key ongoing (as opposed to initial) aspect of organizing the treatment centers on when to use which treatment modality—family versus individual sessions and, when possible, group sessions. We have described in detail the rationale for family sessions. Here, we describe the purpose and place of individual and group sessions in the family-centered relational approach.

Individual Sessions

As we described in Chapter 1, often, especially at the beginning of therapy, the relationship between the child and the nonoffending parent may be quite strained. The parent may be angry with the child, may not believe her, may blame her, and may feel guilty about the abuse. The child may feel frightened of or angry toward the nonoffending parent. As a result, the child may feel too constrained to talk freely in the presence of the parent. Individual sessions with the child allow her to begin to describe her experience and feelings associated with it.

Once the child articulates her feelings, we turn her back to the family and work with her to express herself directly or with our help. Usually, the major work is between mother and daughter. We work with the impact on nonabused siblings of the abuse and events following disclosure in separate sessions, with and without the mother.

Just as there may be reason to meet with the child individually, the parent may have information or feelings that would more appropriately be discussed without the child present. However, we always look for ways to build on the information provided by the parent in these individual sessions to enhance her relationship with her child. Thus, in our approach, we do not generally conduct ongoing, separate, individual therapies with family members, except with the member who offended (discussion to follow). Instead, we use individual sessions of varying length as part of the family therapy.

Individual sessions are useful in the following situations:

1. When a family member indicates, or when we sense, that she or he feels or might feel uncomfortable discussing particular content in front of other family members. For instance, in a first meeting with the mother, if we sense that she is quite angry with the child for disclosing the abuse and that her anger might inhibit the child from speaking to us, we might ask her permission to meet alone with the child the first time, at least for part of the session. In another example, an abused child might directly or indirectly (through body lan-

guage, shyness, etc.) indicate that she is uncomfortable discussing her feelings about her abusive father in front of her mother.

2. When particular contents would be inappropriate to discuss in front of other family members, usually children—for instance, marital issues.

Individual sessions may last anywhere from a few minutes to a full hour, and may occur once, a few times, or be ongoing for several weeks. Although, when the content is appropriate, we generally work toward family members becoming more able to share their experiences directly with one another, individual sessions can serve as a forum in which a family member can initially express and clarify her or his thoughts and feelings, and discuss what makes it difficult to share these with particular family members. These sessions can also be used to explore and try out new ways of interacting. Individual sessions usually end with a Decision Dialogue.

The one area in which we do conduct more ongoing periods of individual therapy is in working with the family member who offended. As we discuss in detail in Chapter 7, the family member who offended is seen individually until he has clearly taken full responsibility for the abuse and has demonstrated empathy for the child he victimized. This series of individual sessions may last from weeks to months. These sessions with the member who offended go on in parallel to the mix of family and individual sessions with the child, nonoffending parent, and siblings, and in some cases, family sessions with the offending member and nonoffending parent (or, in the case of an offending juvenile, with his parents).

Group Sessions

In the context of the relational approach, group sessions among abused children or nonoffending mothers can play several useful functions and provide an excellent forum for implementation of the central treatment principles, including multimodality and information transfer, eliciting stories of pride and "both–and" possibilities, therapy as a collaborative process, and the role of culturally based gender beliefs in creating the possibility of incest. However, despite the tremendous usefulness of groups, they add a level of organizational complexity that is unwieldy for many practicing clinicians, whether working in private practice or in agencies. In fact, it was these organizational issues—such as maintaining a certain size caseload, coordinating family appointments to allow for group to occur on the same day for as many families as possible (because of families' often great difficulties coming to clinic more than once a week), securing rooms, and so forth, that led us to suspend using group therapy. Those interested in the specific ways in which group sessions function within the relational approach can find an extensive discussion in our manual (Fraenkel et al., 1996).

LINKING TREATMENT MODALITIES: THE DECISION DIALOGUE

Basic Concepts

The process of working with the child to determine what to share from an individual session, how, when, and with whom in the family to share it is called the Decision Dialogue. It is essentially a variant of another key collaborative practice, Talking about Talking (discussed next). The difference is that whereas Talking about Talking refers to discussions between the therapist and family members about what to talk about *within* a particular modality, the Decision Dialogue involves talking about the transfer of material *across* therapy modalities. As information is transferred between the modalities, it is enriched and enlarged: Each new telling brings new reactions, new perspectives.

The Decision Dialogue becomes the critical link between two or more modalities. Although we use it to link individual sessions with any family member back to family meetings, it is especially important in bridging individual sessions with the child, because our interest is in strengthening the connections between the child and the nonoffending parent and other family members. Because the child collaborates in deciding with whom to share material about herself, the Decision Dialogue often brings forth issues or feelings that keep her from sharing material with family members (Sheinberg et al., 1994). In other words, when the child does not want to share information, that in itself is revealing to the therapist. These are often the moments when we learn most about problematic aspects of family relationships and are the best source of relational information. We often find that when a child does not wish to talk with a family member, it is because she fears retribution. Understanding this has led to productive exchanges about a child's fear of her parent's anger. In our sessions, nonoffending parents and their children have been able to discuss the "dangers" of talking with each other. With these concerns articulated, the therapist is better able to respond to the relational difficulties that constrain the child from turning toward those family members.

In addition to offering the child and other family members multiple perspectives on their experiences and assisting us to identify problems in family communication, we find that the process of engaging in the Decision Dialogue increases the child's sense of personal agency. Because incest is perpetrated and perpetuated through the person who offended intimidating the child not to tell, engaging the child repeatedly in decisions about what personal material to communicate to others seems to be tremendously empowering.

Guidelines for Practice

Although Decision Dialogues can be carried out with any family member, in most cases, it will be with the child. After commenting on the importance of what the child has said, the therapist initiates the Decision Dialogue by asking her what she thinks about telling other family members this material. For instance, when an abused child reveals a problem in her relationship with her mother during an individual session, the therapist engages her in a dialogue to decide whether, when, and how to bring this problem up with the mother in a family session.

If the child says she would not want to share material in the family session, the therapist explores her reservations and listens especially for indications that the child would not feel safe doing so; in many cases, as noted earlier, the child's reservations center upon the fear of parental retribution. If so, the therapist engages the child in a discussion of what would make her feel safer or more comfortable in sharing this material. Often, the child may need assurances that the parent will not punish her, and the therapist can work out a plan with the child for the therapist to talk with the parent either with or without the child present to set the stage for the child's discussion of this material with the parent or other family members.

Examples

The following vignette is taken from Sheinberg et al. (1994, pp. 268–270). In addition to illustrating the Decision Dialogue in action, it is an excellent demonstration of how a multimodal approach allows themes to emerge in one modality (group) that the child does not yet feel comfortable addressing in another modality (family). Other examples are provided in Chapter 8, in which individual and family therapeutic modalities are discussed.

Dorothy (age 11) was referred to our project after her mother (Anna) discovered her stepfather abusing her. When we first met Dorothy and her mother, Dorothy's stepfather was in jail for having molested her over a period of several years.

In a family session, Anna described her frustration with Dorothy's refusal to talk with her about the abuse and, more generally, with her pattern of beginning to talk, only to abruptly say, "Never mind." When the therapist tried to interact with Dorothy, she, too, found Dorothy reticent to speak. Dorothy responded to questions with "I don't know" or shoulder shrugs. The mother left the family meeting feeling frustrated with her daughter but relieved that the therapist also had a chance to experience their pattern of interaction.

The therapist knew that Dorothy had been left in South America to live with her grandmother when her mother came to the United States, where she married and had two more children. Based on this information, we speculated that while Dorothy wanted to talk with Anna about important matters, she was also fearful that she could not count on her. The pattern that had developed between them seemed to reinforce this fear: As Anna grew increasingly frustrated, Dorothy would withdraw from her.

Based on this observation, we decided to develop a role play in the children's group with the extrapolated theme: "You want to tell your mother something and she won't listen." Dorothy was asked to play her own mother. Becky, another child, was to try to get Dorothy's attention. Jane, a third child, observed and commented on this interaction. With this simple instruction, the children acted out the following scenario:

DOROTHY: (*Spontaneously picks up a play phone and addresses Becky, who is trying to talk to her.*) I told you not to bother me when I'm on the phone. Now go back to bed. It's nine o'clock already and you're not going to wake up tomorrow for school, and I'm going to have problems. Tomorrow, I have a deadline on my job and I have to finish a paper.

JANE: (*Has been observing, spontaneously picks up a paper cup that she uses as a phone.*) You know how children are. Be friendly to her. If she wants to ask you . . .

DOROTHY: (*Speaking into play phone*) She knows that when I'm on the phone, she's not supposed to be asking me questions. She has to wait until I'm finished.

JANE: Yeah, but . . .

DOROTHY: She could tell me tomorrow. Right now, it's past her bedtime and she needs to get her rest, and if she doesn't get her rest, tomorrow morning she's not going to wake up. And I think this is none of your business.

JANE: I know it isn't, but if she wants to ask you an important question, you should listen to her.

DOROTHY: She'll tell me tomorrow.

JANE: Yeah, but if it's important stuff about school or something, you should listen.

DOROTHY: Well, she will tell me tomorrow.

JANE: Oh, while she's going to school?

DOROTHY: Yeah.

JANE: What if you had to go early to work or something and you can't get the information?

DOROTHY: Well, then she'll have to hold it until after school.

JANE: Well, you never know.

DOROTHY: Never know what?

JANE: I don't know, just think about it.

DOROTHY: Think about what?

JANE: Think about what she tells you. She probably got touched or something.

DOROTHY: How do you know?

JANE: I know everything. My daughter had it.

From the role play, the therapist learned about Dorothy's perception of her mother. In a Decision Dialogue session with Dorothy, the therapist expanded on Dorothy's worry about talking with Anna. Dorothy expressed her fear that if she spoke her feelings, they would anger her mother. The therapist helped her to entertain other possible reactions from her mother, and proposed that if Dorothy told Anna just one thing—"Sort of like a little test to see what happened"—she would stop the test if Anna became angry. With this assurance, Dorothy thought a family meeting would be a good idea.

As part of the family session, the therapists—together with the mother and daughter—designed an exercise to address their difficulty. Since both Dorothy and Anna enjoyed art, they designed a card together. Dorothy was instructed to hold up the card whenever she wanted her mother's attention. Anna would indicate when she could listen by holding up her fingers. The effect of the experiment was immediate and dramatic. It transformed a typically painful encounter into a sort of game in which any possible rejection would be of the card, not of Dorothy. It also allowed Anna not to feel pressured and angry.

Mother and daughter began to talk openly about Dorothy's feelings regarding Anna's new boyfriend. Meanwhile, this information was transferred to the caretakers' group, where the adults concentrated on balancing the potential problems of the boyfriend's presence with Anna's need for companionship. With the help of the other mothers, Anna decided to continue her relationship with her boyfriend but to see him outside her home. This relationship was also discussed in a family session with Anna's two younger children present. She was able both to protect her younger children, who were still responding to the loss of their father, and to be open with them about seeing her boyfriend. Though she had previously thought she should not tell the children the truth about where she was when she spent time with her boyfriend, Anna, with the support of the other mothers, was able to reflect on the difference between privacy and secrecy.

In this example, the multimodal program, with its "permeable boundaries," allowed the therapist to abstract a theme from a family meeting and introduce it into the children's group in the form of an activity. The information produced by the activity allowed the therapist both to engage the child in a Decision Dialogue about revealing more of her feelings to her mother and to design a task to change mother and daughter's usual pattern of interacting. Additionally, transferring information to the caretakers' group provided an opportunity for this mother to generate new ideas about meeting her children's needs as well as her own social ones.

Another example of the use of the Decision Dialogue is drawn from the case of Laurie, presented in Chapter 2.

MARCIA: There's something else I want to ask you and it is more complicated. You had a very hard time talking directly to your mother about the abuse. Can you help me understand more about that?

LAURIE: Because I never really talked to my mom about sex. She always told me that when I become a teenager, I should never trust a guy if he says he loves me and cares about me, and then I won't get pregnant. That's the only thing she ever said to me about sex. Also it is strange for me to talk about Tom and what he did, because he was her husband.

MARCIA: Could you say more about that?

LAURIE: I don't know what to say to her. It was her husband, and I don't know what to say to her. Because I do think my mom thinks it is also a little bit my fault.

MARCIA: In what way?

LAURIE: I don't know. I think my mom believes that it's my fault, too. Sometimes I think she thinks that it is my fault because I didn't tell her. But, how was I going to tell her when I was being threatened? I was scared that he would hurt me and my brothers. I also worried that my mom could get hurt.

MARCIA: Is there anything your mom does that makes you think she thinks that it was your fault?

LAURIE: I don't know, but I do think she thinks it's my fault.

MARCIA: When you are grown up, and if you have a little girl, and this happened to her, would you think it was a little bit her fault?

LAURIE: No, because it happened to me, I would not think it was her fault. I would get him out of the house. One day I got angry with my mother and said that she should have known not to marry him, and then none of this would have happened. I said, "it's your fault a little, too." Then I slammed the door like I always do.

MARCIA: Has your mother said anything to you about it being your fault in any way?

LAURIE: I don't think so.

MARCIA: Um-hmm, but you were letting her know how you felt?

LAURIE: Yes, because I do think it is my mother's fault a little, a very little.

MARCIA: Her fault?

LAURIE: Yes, that she married him, but just don't tell my mother I said that.

MARCIA: I won't, If you don't want me to. Why do you not want me to tell her?

LAURIE: Because I guess that she will be mad at me for saying that. She will think that I am mad at her, because I am.

MARCIA: Do you think she's a little mad at herself now?

LAURIE: She says she wishes she could go back to when it didn't happen to me. I told her, "You know, Mom, things will never go back to how they used to be."

MARCIA: Do you think that part of the reason you think she blames you secretly is because you secretly blame her a little bit?

LAURIE: I think so.

MARCIA: Well, I said I am not going to tell her, which I'm not, but maybe we ought to think about you telling her.

LAURIE: Today?

MARCIA: Maybe. I'll tell you why. Let's see if it makes sense to you. I think that if you know that you can talk about whatever feelings and thoughts you have about your mother, the less scared and confused you will feel. See, I think, for instance, you blaming her a little bit is also how she may feel. Also, I don't know that she blames you at all. I really don't know. But if she does, wouldn't it be better if she spoke to you about it? And if she doesn't, wouldn't it be better for you to know that she doesn't? So I am thinking that maybe it would be a good idea for you to talk to her about both things. Why are you smiling?

LAURIE: (*Laughs nervously.*)

MARCIA: What do you think?

LAURIE: I don't know.

MARCIA: What?

LAURIE: It makes me nervous.

MARCIA: Yes.

LAURIE: Because I guess I think she will get mad at me.

MARCIA: Has that happened?

LAURIE: Not really. I don't know, but I think that she will say something to me at home.

MARCIA: Um-hmm.

LAURIE: Like get mad, but I really don't know.

MARCIA: Did that ever happen? Where you said certain things and she got mad?

LAURIE: Well, yes. I remember once my cousin hit me. I am not sure if he was playing or joking around, so I told the social worker and I didn't tell my mom. So when they spoke to my mom, she got angry that I hadn't told her, but I told them.

MARCIA: So you had an experience where in front of people your mom doesn't act angry but at home she gets angry?

LAURIE: Yes.

MARCIA: What if we talk about how you are worried that if you say certain things here, she will act nice, and then when you get home, she might be angry. What if we just talk about that?

LAURIE: OK.

MARCIA: And then, if she reassures you, maybe you can decide whether you want to talk to her about other things.

LAURIE: I think I did tell her once when I was here that I felt it was her fault. A little.

MARCIA: I think you did, actually.

LAURIE: I think I did, too.

MARCIA: I don't think you ever asked her though, if she blames you.

LAURIE: Yes, I know I didn't do that part.

MARCIA: Right.

LAURIE: I think I can talk about that today.

MARCIA: What would you rather talk about?

LAURIE: If she blames me a little.

MARCIA: Also, just in general, that if you say things to her, she will be nice here, and then she will be really mad at you at home?

LAURIE: OK.

MARCIA: Shall we talk about that, too?

LAURIE: Yes.

MARCIA: OK.

CLIENT-DIRECTED SESSIONS: TALKING ABOUT TALKING

Basic Concepts

Related to the Decision Dialogue, Talking about Talking is a practice that engages family members in decisions about the content and flow of sessions as well as reflections upon the process, usefulness, and success of the treatment. Talking about Talking allows for what we call a "client-determined agenda" (Sheinberg et al., 1994). Whereas the Decision Dialogue revolves around determining the flow of information between sessions using different modalities, Talking about Talking centers on determining what gets talked about within any particular session.

The rationale for Talking about Talking is as follows. In a number of treatment programs described in the literature, therapists follow a more or less predetermined format and bring up particular themes in particular sessions (see Hildebrand, 1988; Mandell et al., 1989; Nelki & Walters, 1989). A major rationale for this high degree of structure is that abused children and their family members frequently are quite reluctant to talk about certain aspects of their incest-related experiences, or that they may not realize that some of their feelings, thoughts, and behaviors are common sequelae of incest. Structured programs are designed to ensure that major psychological and social issues found in research to be associated with the incest experience are broached for all children and family members at some point.

Like those clinicians who advocate a more structured format, we recognize the difficulties that abused children (and their families) often have in articulating and understanding aspects of their experience. We, too, are concerned with seeing that abused children have the opportunity to express and deal with all of the issues that pertain to them. However, in the relational approach, ideas and themes associated with the dominant therapy discourse on incest (e.g., shame, guilt, secrecy) are introduced only if the child or another family member has spontaneously provided relevant material. Because our focus is on assisting each child to articulate her unique experience with incest, and the effects of this experience on her self-accounts, we have avoided a format that might at times unwittingly preempt this process and, instead, lead her to view herself in terms of generic assumptions about incest victims; that is, we have been concerned with allowing the child to address incest-relevant issues in her own time and in her own way. We also believe that a more open-ended, flexible format, in which the child determines whether and when certain topics are discussed, avoids another potential problem with more structured formats: that therapists may come to see symptoms or locate feelings in children when they may not exist.

Rather than relying on a structured format and curriculum that include a list of important topics to be discussed, we find that the constant, recursive flow of information across therapeutic modalities ensures that a wealth of feelings, ideas, and perspectives are always available for discussion. The use of family sessions along with individual sessions provides opportunities for the whole range of incest-related issues to emerge and be used in the therapy. Those that are relevant to a particular child and her family at any particular juncture become the focus of the work at that time; when other themes and issues become salient to the child, these are addressed in turn. By allowing the child to select from this flow and to generate the content of sessions, we assist her to take charge of telling her story, enlarging her experience in all its complexity.

Guidelines for Practice

Talking about talking involves three practices:

1. Encouraging family members to participate in setting the therapy agenda
2. Encouraging family members to indicate when they want to switch topics
3. Encouraging family members to comment on the therapy

These are discussed in turn below.

Encouraging Family Members to Participate in Setting the Therapy Agenda

At the beginning of a session, the therapist asks family members what they would like to discuss, indicates any other topics she or he thinks might be important, and decides jointly with family members what topics will be discussed. Oftentimes, the content will have been selected through a Decision Dialogue in a previous session.

Encouraging Family Members to Indicate When They Want to Switch Topics

The therapist attends to the verbal and nonverbal cues (facial expressions, voice tone, gestures) of family members as they talk about a topic, attentive to signs of discomfort. Family members are asked to comment on how they feel talking about the topic, and whether they feel alright about continuing or would like to change topics for a while. If they wish to change topics, the therapist asks what it was that made the topic so uncomfortable, when they believe it may be possible to return to the uncomfortable topic, and what, if anything, might make it easier to talk about it the next time. Especially when talking about the abuse, it is useful to set some kind of time frame around when to return to talking about it—first, so that it does get discussed, and second, so that the family does not misinterpret our encouraging them to take breaks as a sign that we are uncomfortable discussing the abuse. A useful phrase for setting this time frame is, "So why don't we take a break from talking about the abuse and talk about some other things. Before we do, when do you think we could return to talking about the abuse?"

Although this aspect of Talking about Talking is important throughout the therapy, it is particularly important in the beginning, because a major portion of the first session or sessions with the family centers on family members' describing painful events in their lives since disclosure of the abuse, as well as relating the history of the sexual abuse. From the outset, the therapist needs to engage the family in decisions about how much to talk about the abuse at any one time.

Encouraging Family Members to Comment on the Therapy

The therapist asks family members periodically to comment on how they feel the therapy is going as a whole, or, in a particular session, asks them to comment on what has and has not helped them, and what they found interesting or boring, comfortable or uncomfortable, and why. The therapist and family members think and talk about ways to use the family's comments to change how they will work together.

Examples

Prior to asking a family member who offended about the details of his abusive behavior, we ask him if it would be alright to talk about this now, and ask him to tell us if and when it becomes too uncomfortable to continue. Even if he does not directly tell us when he is uncomfortable, we attend to his nonverbal signs (tense facial expressions, down cast eyes, coughs and sighs, long stretches, shifting in seat) and may ask him if it is still OK to ask questions about the abuse. If he says yes, we continue; if he says no, we say this is fine and, together, decide upon another topic. Before leaving the discussion of abuse, we might ask what was it that made this material uncomfortable to discuss. This question often facilitates the offending family member to express emotion (shame, anger, hurt, guilt, sadness, fear), which we validate by saying something to the effect of, "It's often hard to talk about this stuff, and you're doing a good job of it," or some other comment that lets him know he is not alone in his experience of the difficulties in admitting to abusive behavior, and that we appreciate how hard it can be. We also often ask the offending member to tell us when we can ask more questions about the abuse—in a few minutes, in the next session, and so on. Sometimes, especially at the end of a challenging session in which the offending member spoke in some detail about events and feelings, we might emphasize how well he did in facing and discussing these issues and ask him if he feels at all proud of himself for doing so.

We do the same Talking about Talking when we work with the abused child, with her mother, with mother and child together, or with the entire family. Our fundamental stance is that we try to respect the emotional integrity of the individual or family and want to allow family members to protect themselves from questions that feel intrusive or too difficult at the time. In addition to its importance in maintaining a safe therapeutic context, this collaboration around pacing the approach to questions and content allows family members to feel that this is truly their therapy, something they are in charge of, which makes it more likely that they will want to take responsibility for making it successful and to "own" the insights and changes that come about as a result of it.

COAUTHORING DOCUMENTS TO OTHER PROFESSIONALS

Basic Concepts

In addition to collaborating with families around decisions about the flow of topics and information within the therapy context, we also collaborate with them in decisions about the flow of information between the therapy context and larger or "surrounding" systems—child welfare, the courts, physicians, schools, and others involved with the family. We consult with the family to decide how and what to communicate in phone or face-to-face contacts, and we work with them to coauthor official letters to larger systems agencies. Often, these letters are progress reports sent to judges or CPS case managers. Coauthoring these evaluations with the family can have a number of benefits. First, it provides natural and meaningful opportunities for therapist and family to evaluate their work together and to become accountable to each other as well as to the courts. Asking the broad question, "What should we tell them about how far we've gotten in dealing with the abuse?", can lead to an honest appraisal of the work in a practical rather than moralistic tone. This can be especially useful in work with family members who offended. On the one hand, disparities between what the offending family member would *like* to be able to say to the judge versus how far he's actually come in taking responsibility for and understanding the impact of the abuse can dramatically move the therapy forward. On the other hand, where there has been much progress, the ability of the therapist and member who offended to coauthor an honestly positive report can be tremendously rewarding for the member who offended.

Second, rather than aligning him- or herself with the courts and CPS against the family, the therapist can frame the need to write an evaluation as an opportunity for her or him and the family to report on their *shared* work. This can strengthen the therapist's relationship with the family, without forming a coalition between her or him and the family against the regulatory agencies (Imber-Black, 1988).

Guidelines for Practice: Example

The following case vignette richly describes the process and benefits of coauthoring with the family documents to other professionals and organizations, in this case, child welfare.

A Latino family of nine sought therapy because they believed it would help them win back their four daughters who were in foster care. An earlier charge of sexual abuse against their teenage son had been dropped, but an accompanying charge of neglect against the parents was not. Foster placement was continued because child welfare and the psychiatrist evaluating two of the girls determined that the parents were generally irresponsible and uncooperative. (The boys had also been placed but ran away to their parents and were allowed to remain at home.) The parents had refused to acknowledge that they had behaved irresponsibly with their children. Furthermore, they had instructed their children not to talk about the family, warning them that it would postpone their return home. This was especially alarming to child welfare and the evaluating psychiatrist. The cycle of interaction that developed between the parents and the professionals was a classic "game without end." The more the parents felt accused, the less they cooperated; the less they cooperated, the more convinced the professionals became that they could not return the children until the parents were more cooperative and learned parenting skills.

At the time we met the family members, they were in an elaborate struggle with all the professionals involved. Because the family found the Ackerman Clinic through a friend, we expected that the family would be more open to a relationship with us. However, the parents stated unequivocally that they were only coming to therapy because they were told it would help them get their children back.

Our first step was to address our relationship with child welfare. At a meeting with a child welfare worker and supervisor, together with the family, we sought to define a therapy contract based on the family's stated needs. We were moderately successful in that the parents said they thought that therapy might help their sons deal with the trauma of being removed from the home. Since the boys' return, they were experiencing sleep disturbances, bowel difficulties, and fear about being removed again. Once we had invited the family to describe their concerns, we began to hear the family members' story of the "abuse" they received from the system. Inquiry about the history of these feelings elicited stories of the parents' own removal from their homes as children, which had clearly influenced their present behavior. Ms. A had been taken from her home after her mother left her children alone for three days. Mr. D had been sent away to a residential school because his father, who did not understand English, couldn't advocate to keep him at home. Both parents were determined to fight for the return of their children and protect them as they believed their parents had not done for them.

Ironically, the parents deeply believed that acknowledgment of any "wrongdoing" would threaten the return of their children, while the regulatory agency (child welfare) held this as a criterion for change—an expression of responsibility—that would lead to the return of the children to their parents. Against this background, the letter that child welfare required from us provided a vehicle for a conversation between us and the family outside the parameters of the struggle.

We invited the parents to join us in writing the report. They described their feelings about their children, their children's needs, and how they intended to meet those needs. Future planning was substituted for recriminations over past behavior. This orientation allowed us to ask the parents to anticipate how their future behavior with the children would be different from the past. With little hesitation, the parents spoke about the need to be sure that the children attended school regularly, the desirability of keeping their arguments from the children, and the need to be more discriminating in the movies they rented for their children.

Together, in front of a word processor, the parents and therapist worked on phrasing these thoughts. Woven into this task were conversations about the nature of the parents' fights and child welfare's accusations of irresponsibility, as well as frank discussion about whether child welfare was accurate in its assessment. Because the frame was the future, and they could participate in how the letter was authored, the past became a point of departure rather than a painful story etched in stone.

The openness of the dialogue revealed an unresolved and festering conflict: Ms. A wanted to be legally married and Mr. D refused. Once the couple broached this issue, the therapeutic inquiry shifted to the way in which household decisions were made. What emerged was that both Ms. A and Mr. D assumed that he was the authority on matters of family life. As these ideas were expressed, Ms. A became increasingly open with us about her fears and desires. Mr. D began to explore the ways in which he associated his masculinity with being "the boss."

The coauthoring experience seemed to produce an observable change in the couple's pattern of interacting with the judicial system and CPS, as well as with each other. Child welfare eventually recommended that the children return home but insisted on a transitional plan in which, for 2 months, the children would spend only weekends at home. Ms. A spent several days writing her own letter detailing why the plan was misguided. The parents had found a new way to fight for their children. Ms. A told us: "Now I am more professional, more effective. I don't yell and scream or just stop talking. Now I calmly stand up for myself."

The coauthored letter provided a way of addressing the either–or dilemma of social control versus therapy. Coauthoring the requisite report and addressing the future rather than the past created a shift in perspective for both the family and the therapist, from which a new description of therapy could evolve. The consideration of questions in the letter writing process helped change the context from one in which the therapist felt constrained and the parents felt judged, to one in which the therapist felt "freed" and the parents felt accepted. As the relationship between the therapist and family became more collaborative, the couple began to develop their own new ideas about how to parent. Once Ms. A had shared her frustration about her relationship with Mr. D, the therapist broadened the conversation to include ideas about power differentials between men and women.

SUMMARY

In this chapter, we have described specific collaborative practices for working with families in which sexual abuse has occurred. These practices center around decisions regarding organizing the treatment, choosing when to use which treatment modality, transferring information between modalities, creating a client-centered agenda in session, and communicating with the other professionals involved with the family. As we have illustrated, the process of therapists engaging in these collaborative decisions with families often has the additional effect of stimulating more open communication and collaboration among family members. However, family members, especially nonoffending parents, sometimes begin therapy with a variety of beliefs and feelings that challenge their ability to connect with other family members, particularly the abused child. In Chapter 6, we discuss practices that assist nonoffending mothers to understand and overcome issues that limit their capacity to support and protect their abused daughters.

Chapter Six

Strengthening Safe Family Relationships

In Chapters 4 and 5, we described several therapeutic foci and practices that directly or indirectly help to strengthen the child's safe family relationships. For instance, helping the child and nonoffending family members acknowledge their often-secret attachments and loyalties to the person who offended is essential to clarifying which relationships can be safely maintained and strengthened and which cannot. Other relationship-building practices discussed earlier include locating sources of pride, often submerged by the incest story; and building family members' sense of agency and choice through collaborative therapeutic practices such as the Decision Dialogue and Talking about Talking. Especially with these latter practices, the child becomes empowered to control how and what she talks about with other family members. When the Decision Dialogue reveals that the child feels uncomfortable speaking to her mother or other nonoffending caretakers about something, we can identify and work on the behaviors and premises that block their communication and connection.

In this chapter, we approach strengthening the child's family relationships by focusing on work with the nonoffending mother that facilitates her connection to the child and her own coming to terms with the abuse. In our professional workshops, we are often asked how to work with mothers who do not (or initially did not) believe their child was abused; mothers who are angry at or rejecting of the child; and mothers who describe or demonstrate a lack of warmth or affection for the child. This chapter describes how the relational approach deals with these challenging issues.

We describe the work as occurring in individual sessions with the mother, because, at the very least, when other family members are not involved (or not available), the therapy will most often include the mother and child. However, the points and practices recommended here can be applied in individual sessions with other nonoffending adult family members who may have issues similar to those of the parent. These points can also be applied to family sessions with two or more nonoffending adults.

Exploration of the issues described in this section is usually best *initiated* without the abused child present, both in order to free the parent up to discuss the issues fully and to avoid exposing the child to the adults' thoughts and feelings that might be upsetting for the child to hear. Once these feelings and beliefs are discussed and better understood, the therapist may engage the parent or other adult family members in a Decision Dialogue about what to communicate from these sessions to the child, and how best to do so. As the parent resolves issues that made it difficult to feel close to her child, she may feel more pride in herself; as she comes to terms with the abuse and feels greater self-confidence, she may be better able to feel close and protective toward her child.

Each parent will bring her own particular psychological and interpersonal issues to therapy. Some of these issues may relate directly to the events surrounding and including the abuse of her child; others may predate the abuse and be renewed or exacerbated, or be relatively unaffected by it. Some parents may have fairly intensive, extensive, and/or long-standing problems; others may have few or none. Therefore, we cannot present a conclusive list of issues and approaches to working with the parent, especially in terms of the preexisting problems she may bring to therapy. Rather, we outline the most frequent issues presented by parents. It is not necessary to address all or even any of the following issues with all parents. Keeping in mind the notion of the "client-determined agenda," the point is to be aware of the following possible issues and allow each parent the opportunity to raise her concerns rather than imposing upon her a predetermined agenda.

DIFFICULTIES IN BEING CLOSE TO THE CHILD

Some parents describe difficulties feeling or showing warmth and affection toward their children, especially toward the abused child. When they describe this as a problem that predated disclosure of the child's abuse, the parent's self-blame may center upon the idea that if she had been closer to her child, the abuse would never have occurred. In other cases, the mother reports that the distance between herself and her daughter began, or became much worse, following the abuse.

Three approaches are particularly useful in working with the mother's sense of distance from her daughter:

1. Exploring the attachment to the person who offended—loyalty binds
2. Exploring the mother's gender premises—especially beliefs about whether the needs of men and boys take precedence over those of women and girls, including the need for protection and sexual expression
3. Exploring the mother's relationship with her own mother

Because previous chapters have described in detail working with attachments and resulting loyalty binds, this chapter focuses on the latter two issues.

Basic Concepts

Exploring the Mother's Gender Premises

In some cases, the nonoffending parent's difficulty being close and supportive toward her (female) abused child is due to unarticulated beliefs about what boys (or men) need in terms of emotional protection versus what girls (or women) need, as well as beliefs about what is normal sexual behavior for boys and men versus girls and women. The nonoffending parent of a child abused by her brother or cousin (or young uncle) may be more concerned about the stress that the disclosure of and punishment for incest will cause for the boy who offended than about the effects of incest upon the abused girl. The parent in this case may believe that male sexuality by nature requires the boy or man to pursue and seduce the woman with unbridled confidence; that it is natural for boys (or men) to make mistakes and get confused in dealing with their arousal, and that these mistakes should not be severely punished; or that what the offending boy or man did was just a more extreme version of "normal" sexual play; and so on. Especially in the case of a juvenile who has offended, the parent may be concerned that punishment of his behavior will wreck his sexual self-confidence or change his sexual orientation toward homosexuality, which for some parents is a concern.

In addition, the parent might believe that girls and women are stronger than boys and men, are better able to deal with stress, and that therefore, the offending boy's emotional needs should be given precedence over the girl's. As a result, the parent may attempt to protect him from any negative consequences or feelings, even at the risk of neglecting the girl's well being.

In some cases, the nonoffending parent or some other adult family member may hold the belief that girls (and women in general) are by nature sexually seductive, and that the abused girl somehow stimulated, teased, led on, or otherwise elicited the boy's or man's sexual actions toward her.

Guidelines for Practice

These and other beliefs about differences between the sexes in what they can endure, what they need, and what they are entitled to regarding sex, sexual misbehavior, and emotional protection are best explored with the nonoffending parent (and other nonoffending adults) with an attitude of respectful curiosity. At the same time, the therapist can introduce alternative perspectives that embody greater fairness and justice between the sexes; can explore the differences and overlaps between these perspectives and those of the family members; and discuss the relative strengths and problems of the different perspectives, especially in terms of the adult family members' ability fully to protect the abused child in the future.

Example

In one family, a mother, June, described how she had cautioned her daughter never to trust boys. She clearly believed that girls need to protect themselves and had warned her daughter never to take off her panties or accept bribes for sexual behavior. June was particularly adamant about this because her older sister had been abused by a favorite uncle. To June's horror, her daughter was abused by a teenage neighbor, the older brother of her daughter's close playmate.

As June recounted the discovery of the abuse, she kept angrily interjecting how she had warned her daughter to be careful, with the implication that the daughter was at fault for the abuse. The therapist listened and encouraged June to describe all the reasons she had learned not to trust men, how women and girls must protect themselves, and so on.

After this full elaboration of her beliefs and the experiences behind them, the therapist gently asked if June had ever experienced times when she felt more positively about men. Slowly, June began to recount different experiences, although events that began positively often ended with sadness, hurt and disappointment. Especially painful was the time June had allowed herself to believe that her daughter's father loved her and would marry her if she became pregnant. She described her shock and confusion when he betrayed her by leaving her before the baby was even born, and how she had struggled as a single parent. She was particularly angry for allowing herself to be "duped."

Gradually, the therapist introduced questions that brought forth June's fortitude, integrity, and determination. June began to see herself as someone who on occasion made poor choices, and as someone also whom she liked and respected. Following this focus on herself, a more complex and accepting description of her daughter emerged.

Basic Concepts

Exploring the Mother's Own Relationship with Her Mother

In some cases, the nonoffending parent will describe herself as generally "unaffectionate" or even "cold" emotionally, especially toward her child. Exploration of the mother's childhood and adult relationship with her own mother may reveal that she is in some way replicating in her current family a triangle or other pattern from her family of origin. Some examples include the following: (1) She was one of many siblings and never felt particularly cared about by her own mother; (2) she felt left out of her mother and father's (or other mate of the mother's) very exclusive relationship; (3) she was much closer to her father than to her mother, and saw herself as the father's emotional support and confidant when the parents' marital relationship unraveled; (4) she was the *mother's* emotional support, and never wanted to put her own daughter in that difficult position, and so has kept her distance; and/or (5) she was the major caretaker of the other children (or adults) in the family.

These are only a sample of intergenerational scripts found in work with mothers who have reported difficulties feeling close to their daughters (see also Gelinas, 1988). The point here is that it is often fruitful to find a historical explanation of the nonoffending parent's difficulties with closeness.

Guidelines for Practice

After exploring these patterns, it is useful to ask the mother, "How would you have wanted your mother to have parented you?" or "How would you imagine your life to be if your mother had parented you differently?" and to see if there are ways in which the mother can put these wishes or fantasies for herself into action between herself and her own daughter. To encourage this, the therapist might suggest that by changing how she is with her own daughter, she might in some way make peace with what she missed from her own mother. Another way to put this is that families evolve over generations, with each generation having the opportunity to improve upon the last, and that this might be just such an opportunity for herself and her family. In addition, the therapist might bring in the notion that for the mother to be able to become close with her daughter despite her lack of a model from her own childhood (and based only on her imagination of what would have been better for her) might become a source of pride for her.

Example

A mother and her 12-year-old daughter, who had been abused by her step-father, had developed an escalating pattern in which the daughter would seek attention from the mother, who would respond by withdrawing, eventually leading to misbehavior by the daughter that was punished by the mother. The mother partially blamed her daughter for the cycle—she viewed her as insatiable and spoiled—and partially blamed herself, regarding herself as "cold" by nature and incapable of giving her child affection. In addition to being a frustrating interaction in its own right, this pattern kept mother and daughter generally distant, which prevented the daughter from openly discussing her feelings about the abuse. This distance also represented a significant risk factor for the daughter in the future, in that she was not inclined to discuss her concerns with her mother.

The therapist assisted the family to change this pattern by first exploring with the mother, in an individual session, the relationship between her reactions to her daughter and her childhood experiences with her own mother. She reported that she was one of several siblings and had received little affection from her mother. She had always wished she had been closer to her mother and now felt that she, unfortunately, took after her in how she was responding to her daughter. The therapist also helped the mother recognize that she was not always "cold"—that there had been many times when she had reacted warmly toward her daughter, and that she had enjoyed these times.

Although the mother now had greater insight about her reactions, she still believed that it would be difficult to break the pattern with her daughter, because, in the moment, she found her daughter's childish attention-seeking behavior irritating. The therapist suggested that in these moments, she could repeat to herself a "mantra," a simple phrase that could help her see the situation differently and guide her to react differently (see Sheinberg & Penn, 1991, for a more detailed discussion of the use of mantras in family therapy). The therapist suggested the following mantra: "I am going to try to love my daughter the way I wanted to be loved by my own mother."

At the same time, the therapist met individually with the daughter and explored what differences she wanted in her relationship with her mother. Her main wish was to "have more fun" with her mother. She identified one activity with her mother that would represent the beginning of having more fun—going out to dinner. In a Decision Dialogue, the therapist and child discussed how to present this idea to her mother. The mother was then invited into the session to discuss the "fun plan."

At the next appointment, 1 week later, mother and daughter reported, in both individual and family sessions, that they had followed through with all the suggested activities, and that their relationship had improved dramatically. The mother had repeated the mantra daily and found it helped her look at herself and her relationship with her daughter differently—among other things, as an opportunity for her own healing, and not as a burden and reminder of the emotional deprivation she experienced as a child.

PARENTING BELIEFS THAT INTERFERE WITH SUPPORTING THE CHILD

Basic Concepts

In some families, the mother's beliefs about how best to respond to problem behavior and negative events involving the child—even when the child did not cause these events or initiate the behavior—make it difficult for the mother to respond empathically and supportively. A vicious cycle often quickly ensues in which the parent's punitive response leads the child to fear speaking further to her mother about the abuse; the child may then speak with someone else, who tells the mother, who then punishes the child for not speaking with her directly, and the cycle of alienation spirals.

The therapist needs to explore the mother's parenting beliefs and their basis in her family and culture of origin, to reflect with the parent about how her current parenting approach has the unintended impact of pushing the child away; and to invite the parent to consider alternative parenting styles that would work equally well to guide the child's behavior, while at the same time strengthening rather than weakening the parent–child bond.

Guidelines for Practice: Examples

A 6-year-old boy had been abused by a 9-year-old cousin for over 3 years. When his mother discovered the abuse, she described becoming so distraught that she spanked her son for not having told her. The mother reported that in her family and country of origin, spanking was viewed as an acceptable form of punishment, albeit one she used infrequently. In fact, since her discovery of the abuse, she had not spanked the son again.

Although concerned about the negative impact of the mother hitting the son, we did not wish to challenge outright the validity of her parenting beliefs or practices. Instead, in our conversations with her, we expressed concern that her spanking the son might inhibit him from confiding in her in the future. We also wondered aloud if the combination of having been sexually abused, and then hit for not telling, might negatively affect his sense of bodily integrity. She said these points made sense. In the next session with mother and son, she told him she decided that she would no longer hit him, and he smiled and hugged her. She asked him if he thought he would be able to speak more freely to her, knowing now that he wouldn't be physically punished, and he said yes. This emotional exchange began to strengthen their bond.

In another family, a little girl found herself literally unable to speak about her abusive stepfather in her mother's presence. Although her silence was determined by several factors, one reason was that she anticipated criticism from her mother, by whom she frequently felt belittled even prior to disclosure of the abuse. In a joint session with daughter and mother, we identified and communicated the daughter's general expectation that she would be criticized and how it prevented her from speaking openly and trusting her mother. The mother, who up to this point viewed her critical comments as attempts to help her daughter grow up well, had never considered how these comments might interfere with their closeness. With a new understanding of the relational effects of criticism, she found other ways to encourage her daughter's development. At first cautiously, then with eagerness, the daughter opened up to her mother.

WORKING WITH THE NONOFFENDING PARENT'S DENIAL OF THE ABUSE: THE "WHAT IF" DIALOGUE

Basic Concepts

In some families, the nonoffending parent (and/or other nonoffending family members) may deny the facts of the abuse (Trepper & Barrett, 1989). One of the most effective means of encouraging family members to face the abuse more directly is to encourage a "what if" dialogue, a discussion about how the family would be affected "if" the abuse had occurred. This approach can also be used when the abuse has been medically and legally confirmed, and family members agree that the child was abused but deny that the child's sexual abuse was perpetrated by a family member; instead, it might be attributed to a stranger—such as a janitor at school, a babysitter, and so on. (This type of denial is more frequent the younger the child; once the child is old enough to clearly report what happened, it becomes less possible to lay blame elsewhere.)

Guidelines for Practice

The "what if" dialogue can allow the nonoffending parent and other family members to discuss all anticipated aspects of the impact of the hypothetical abuse (or of fully acknowledging that the reported abuse occurred), including the following:

Legal, Social, Financial, and Lifestyle Impact

The therapist explores family members' beliefs regarding the legal impact of the abuse (on the offending person, or possibly the nonoffending parent), the social impact (e.g., potential stigmatization, rejection by extended family and neighbors), and the financial and lifestyle impact (due to loss of income if the offending parent goes to prison, possibly requiring the family to relocate).

Impact on Fundamental Assumptions

The therapist explores family members' beliefs about the impact of the abuse, or of acknowledging it, on fundamental assumptions about themselves in the world in general (e.g., that the world is a just, safe place, where people you love and trust do not harm you or those you love), and about their family and family members in particular (e.g., "John is a good man—he wouldn't do this sort of thing").

Impact on Family Members' Feelings and Loyalties

The therapist explores family members' expectations about what the impact of the abuse might be on how they would feel about each other, especially the types of loyalty binds they would experience. For example, a parent might anticipate feeling unable simultaneously to love the offending son *and* love the abused daughter, and so might deny the abuse altogether in order to avoid confronting her loyalty bind. The therapist might ask, "Could you find a way to continue to love both your children even if one abused the other?"

Gender Premises: Differential Impact and Responsibility for Men/Boys versus Women/Girls

Gender premises can also be examined using the "what if" dialogue. For instance, the therapist could ask: "If your son/husband really had abused your daughter, how do you think it would have happened—who would have started it? Who would be responsible for it, if anyone? How do you think it would have been kept a secret this long? How would your son/husband be affected if the abuse were brought to light? How do you think your daughter would be feeling? What would the appropriate consequences be for your son/husband?" And so on.

By listening carefully to family members' explanations of the hypothetical abuse, the therapist can get a better sense of their underlying gender beliefs and reflect these back in the form of further questions, such as the following, posed to the mother: "I'm noticing that as you talk about who would be affected more, it sounds like you might worry most about how it would have affected your son to have the abuse disclosed; and that you think your daughter would have gotten over it pretty well on her own. Does this fit with your ideas? What are the ways in which you think girls are stronger than boys in general? How about ways in which boys are stronger than girls?" After some discussion of the mother's beliefs, the therapist might ask, "How do you think you came by those ideas?"

Expectations about How the Family Would Cope

In addition to exploring family members' fears and biases regarding the hypothetical abuse, the therapist might ask them to reflect upon how they believe they would cope, individually and as a family, if the abuse were acknowledged as real. How do they believe they would respond to the needs of the abused child? To each others' emotional upset? To further contacts with representatives of the legal system (assuming they've already had such contact—hence, their being in treatment)? What particular individual and family strengths and psychosocial resources could be mobilized in coping with this event? Such a discussion can result in lowering or eliminating altogether the family's denial of the abuse, as they come to see that their existing coping abilities are adequate; or through the discussion, develop a sense of how to enhance their coping abilities in a way that would enable them to face the abuse fully.

Facilitating the Process of "What If" Dialogues

So far, we have focused upon the content of the "what if" dialogue. Three aspects influence the *process* of the dialogue.

1. *Using Talking about Talking.* Family members are likely to feel safer and more in control if the therapist makes ample use of Talking about Talking by asking them how they feel talking about this material, is sensitive to nonverbal cues of discomfort, allows them to switch topics when it becomes too challenging, and decides together with the family when it would be possible to return to the "what if" dialogue. In other words, the therapist should invite the family to codirect the pace and content of the discussion.

2. *Acknowledging family members for their participation.* During this often-delicate discussion of denial, family members may feel encouraged to continue the dialogue about abuse if the therapist acknowledges from time to time how well they're doing discussing this difficult, upsetting material. This can be one of those challenging moments for the therapist, who at some level may feel troubled by the nonoffending parents' seeming unwillingness to accept the facts or impact of the abuse. Yet it is especially important during this phase of the work to remain empathic to the psychological and relational vulnerabilities of these family members that have led them to take a stance of denial, even as the therapist works toward the goal of the family's full recognition of the abuse.

3. *Engaging family members in both–and thinking.* Throughout the "what if" dialogue, the therapist can encourage family members to lower their denial by considering "both–and" possibilities. For example, in a "what if" dialogue with the mother of a bright, talented, generally responsible 19-year-old son who allegedly had abused his 4-year-old sister, the mother said that if her son had truly abused her daughter, she would see him as sick and evil, and could have nothing more to do with him.

The therapist asked a series of questions to assist her to entertain a both–and perspective, such as: "Would it be possible to see your son as having done something terribly wrong, something that might even indicate that he has certain psychological problems, and at the same time, still remember that he is a young man with tremendous gifts and strengths—strengths that might actually help him not do such things in the future? Could you still love him and at the same time hate what he did? Could he possibly basically be a sane person, and yet have done something crazy?" These and other both–and questions allowed the mother to loosen the either–or ways of thinking about her son and the abuse, eventually leading her to consider more directly the possibility that he had abused her daughter.

From a theoretical perspective, working with the family's denial is an excellent example of how all three basic perspectives included in the relational approach—social constructionism, systems, and feminism—work together to provide a balanced, complete intervention. The social constructionist lens provides awareness of the impact of the shameful, fragmenting story of the abuse on the family's identity. "Denial" can be understood through this lens as a response to the family's terror of what it would mean to acknowledge and accept the incest story. In the ways described earlier, the therapist needs to help the family take control of the process of considering this story in their lives, and to counterbalance it with recognition of the more positive stories of pride. Systems theory contributes ideas about the need to explore loyalty binds, intergenerational and cultural sources of beliefs about gender, responsibility, sexuality, and need for care that result in denial. And feminism contributes the moral imperative to move the family beyond denial and into recognition of the abuse and of the very real power differences among family members of different genders that facilitated the abuse.

As family members engage in a detailed consideration of their feelings and thoughts about a hypothetical abuse and their potential coping responses, they may become more comfortable with the possibility of discussing the actual abuse. Their increased comfort with the topic not only may be a result of communicating openly with one another in a safe context, but also may result from the opportunity to see that the therapist does not respond in a harsh, judgmental, moralistic manner. Rather, the therapist models a nonjudgmental curiosity, an interest in each family member's perspective, and supports their strengths as individuals and as a family.

WORKING WITH THE NONOFFENDING PARENT'S HISTORY OF CHILDHOOD SEXUAL ABUSE OR ADULT RAPE

Basic Concepts

In some families, the nonoffending parent may herself have been a victim of sexual abuse or other violence perpetrated by men. She may have a history of childhood sexual abuse, or she may have been raped as an adult. She may also have been physically abused or intimidated by the man who abused her child. In all instances, there are two issues to consider:

1. Her need for individual sessions
2. The impact of her own abuse experience on her ability to comfort and protect the child

Guidelines for Practice

Individual Sessions

In some cases, the child's abuse may have triggered long-forgotten memories of abuse or stimulated emotions associated with "long-remembered" abuse that the parent has never come to terms with or even discussed with anyone, or that she has discussed (or even worked on in previous therapy) but that now trouble her again. As a result, she may need a series of her own individual sessions. The Decision Dialogue can be used to transfer material from the parent's individual sessions to family sessions when such transfer would be useful and appropriate.

Impact of the Mother's Abuse Experience on Her Ability to Comfort and Protect the Child

In some ways, when the parent has herself been abused, she may have a special degree of empathy for what her child has experienced. On the other hand, the parent may confuse her own experience with that of the child or assume she knows what her daughter needs rather than really attending to her child's communications of her needs. In addition, mothers who themselves have been abused as children may experience a particularly high degree of shame and self-blame about their own children's abuse. They may note how terrible they feel that the one thing they vowed would never happen to their own child has happened. The key to working with such mothers is to be particularly gentle and supportive, and to assist them to distinguish between their own and their children's experience of abuse.

The therapist might start this process by working with the mother to identify the aspects of her daughter's abuse that she feels are similar to her own experience, and then move to aspects that she thinks might be different. If she is convinced that the experiences are essentially identical, the therapist might suggest that the next session with the daughter focus upon the mother asking questions that really test this idea and attempt to find out much more about the daughter's unique experience.

The goal of this part of the work is to help the mother separate her own abuse history from that of her daughter, so that she can effectively comfort and protect her daughter. The importance of the mother being able to do this, so that the child feels free to discuss her own experience, is well illustrated by the following case vignette, taken from Sheinberg et al. (1994, pp. 270–271).

Example

Alison, age 8, was referred to the project after disclosing sexual abuse by her paternal uncle. Her parents (Joan and Ben) responded protectively toward Alison by prosecuting Ben's brother and seeking therapy for the family. In initial meetings, Joan revealed that she not only felt enraged and betrayed, but she was also reminded of having been abused during her own childhood. In family meetings, Alison appeared distant and unavailable. In the children's group, she was also noticeably quiet. By contrast, in the mothers' group, Joan was very vocal in discussing how important it was for her child to confront abuse: "I think she needs to get it out, to get it off her chest, at least to tell somebody what happened. When I reached out to tell somebody, there was nobody to tell. I wanted to tell my mother everything, but she wouldn't listen. I kept a lot inside and that's why I think she needs to get it off her chest."

Immediately following disclosure, Alison had talked with her mother about what had happened, and Joan shared with her daughter her own experience of being abused. Over time, however, Alison became reluctant to talk with her mother. At the same time, Alison had difficulty concentrating on her schoolwork and increasingly wet her bed. Joan believed her daughter's concentration was being interrupted by disturbing thoughts of her abuse. Alison had told her mother that, whenever she was quiet, she would remember what her uncle had done to her. Joan asked that the therapist see her daughter individually.

Because Alison was unable to talk directly about her experience, the therapist used what Joan had told her to construct a story about a little girl who could not sit still because of "bad memories." Alison said, "That sounds like me." Alison told the therapist she believed that her mother had forgotten what she had told her about the abuse. When the therapist initi-ated a Decision Dialogue to see if Alison would like to meet with her mother and find out what she remembered, Alison enthusiastically agreed. When asked if she would like her father to be there as well, Alison said she wanted to meet with her mother alone.

The therapist wondered if Alison had felt her mother's story of abuse overshadowed her own experience. In sessions with mother and daughter together, the therapist asked what it would be like for them to hear each other's stories. Alison expressed her concern that if she retold her story, her mother would recall her own experience, which would upset Joan. This provoked a discussion between mother and daughter about how Joan had been able to manage her upset feelings and solve her own difficulties with intrusive thoughts. The therapist asked Alison if she wanted to learn how her mother had been able to do this. When Alison answered affirmatively, Joan offered her daughter potential solutions. With Alison's permission, Joan went on to describe the abuse she had experienced. With the thera-pist's guidance, Joan underscored the differences between their experiences as well as the similarities. The session concluded with mother and daughter deciding to discuss these observations with Alison's father.

In this example, the multimodal aspect of the relational approach al-lowed Joan to initiate an individual session for Alison in which she was able to articulate her fears about her relationship with her mother. Once Alison described her concerns to the therapist, she began to feel confident about sharing more of herself with her mother.

The results in this instance were dramatic. Alison's school perfor-mance improved markedly, her "flashbacks" diminished, and her bed-wet-ting decreased. The child who had described herself as dumb told her mother that she was now a good student. Furthermore, as an outgrowth of discussions in the mothers' group, Joan sought opportunities to relate to Alison in areas other than the abuse. She decided it was important that they not develop a bond exclusively around this shared experience.

LIMITATIONS OF THERAPY

Although the relational approach can be highly effective in strengthening bonds between alienated mothers and daughters, therapy does not always work and is not always possible even to start. For a wide variety of reasons, some mothers are not able, even with professional help, to provide a consistently supportive and protective environment for their children in the immediate present or near future. In these instances (unusual in our experience), children may be separated, at least temporarily, from their mothers. However, as others have advocated (Colapinto, 1995; Minuchin, Colapinto, & Minuchin, 1998), this separation need not become a complete cutoff. Even when children are placed by social services and the mother attends parenting classes, the therapist can continue to see the family and work in the ways described in this chapter.

In some families, the mother is not willing or available for treatment. The therapist must then work with the extended family and/or other caretakers with whom the child lives to strengthen their relationships. Discussions and rituals can be included that allow the child to talk about her feelings for the absent mother, and that help her caretakers accept those feelings.

For example, we saw a family (described briefly in Chapter 1) in which a 6-year-old child was sexually inappropriate with her 5-year-old sibling. It was suspected that both children had been sexually abused by the biological mother's boyfriend. Shortly after this suspicion arose, the mother, who was addicted to crack cocaine, abandoned them and disappeared. For about 1 year, the girls lived with their paternal grandmother, until she suddenly died of heart failure. The children then went to live with their father, his new wife, and their infant son. The young wife was quite alarmed by the girls' sexual activity and responded by punishing them. Furthermore, based on her own history of parental loss and her insecurities about being their "new mother," she would not tolerate any expressions of missing their "undeserving" parent.

In addition to addressing these feelings and ideas in conversations with the parents, the therapist suggested a simple ritual. The family would light three candles once a week: one for the past, one for the present, and one for the future. The ritual helped the stepmother because it prescribed a contained time to tolerate the memories of past family relationships—the children's as well as her own. It created a relational bridge, placing the past in the perspective of a different future that this new blended family was building together, and included the stepmother in the children's memories of their past. As the family members performed this ritual together, they saw that the love, joy, anger, and sadness of the past did not compete with their new life. For the children, it helped them honor their past and their many feelings, and look forward to a different, more secure future.

SUMMARY

In this chapter, we discussed the challenges of working with nonoffending family members, particularly mothers, so as to strengthen their protective relationship with the abused child. We examined gender premises, parenting beliefs, and family-of-origin experiences that may keep a mother disconnected from her child. We introduced a dialogic practice that brings forth the relational fears behind family members' denial of the abuse. And we addressed the ways in which a mother's own history of sexual abuse and trauma may influence her capacity to assist in her child's recovery. Throughout, the core principles and practices were emphasized, such as both–and thinking, the Decision Dialogue and Talking about Talking, the need to recognize and build upon strengths, and the need to locate unrecognized relational meanings that block more satisfying and protective relationships. In Chapter 7, we turn our attention to an equally challenging aspect of the work: treatment of the offending family member.

Chapter Seven

Relational Treatment of Family Members Who Abuse

This chapter describes the relational approach to treatment of family members who have sexually abused another family member. Like others working in this area (Bengis, 1997; Elms, 1990; Jenkins, 1990; Longo, Bays, & Bear, 1996; Ryan & Lane, 1997; Trepper & Barrett, 1989), our emphasis is on helping the offending person to assume responsibility and develop empathy. Relational treatment of persons who offend revolves around the same basic principles and practices that guide treatment of the abused child and nonoffending family members. However, due to the ongoing risks that all who have offended present to family members and possibly other persons, the issue of whom it is appropriate to treat and with what type of treatment must be carefully considered first. We begin with a discussion of these treatment selection issues.

SELECTING THE CORRECT TREATMENT

The clinical and research literature to date suggest that men who sexually abuse children[1] generally require highly specialized assessment and treatment centering on cognitive-behavioral techniques (Maletzky, 1991; Marshall, Laws, & Barbaree, 1990; Murphy & Smith, 1996; Salter, 1988; Schwartz & Cellini, 1995). Therapists not well versed in these therapies must refer persons for such assessment and treatment. We typically refer such men for treatment to an agency or to other professionals with whom we have developed a working relationship.

However, before referring them out, the therapist may be able to work with offending adults to help them assume complete responsibility for the abuse and to develop empathy for the abused child and other family members. Although these treatment goals are included in many cognitive-behavioral treatment protocols, much of the work of cognitive-behavioral-based treatment centers around attempts to change the offending man's sexual interests (from children to adult partners) and to help him master impulse control strategies. Therefore, the unique contribution of the relational approach can be to help the offending family member understand both the relational meanings and motivations behind his abusive behavior, as well as its relational impact. Recognition of these relational causes and effects often motivates the offending person to seek further specialized treatment, whereas he might have been less inclined to do so prior to understanding the meaning and family impact of the abuse.

For example, with one offending adult with whom we worked prior to referring him to specialized treatment, exploration of his family-of-origin experiences revealed that as a young boy, he had witnessed his mother becoming drunk, falling onto the bed, and having intercourse with different partners. He felt both aroused and ashamed watching, and described feeling erotically stimulated much of the time thereafter. In addition, he later revealed that he had been molested as a young teen by an older female cousin in an incident that he had never disclosed. Whereas, at the onset of our work together, he denied abusing his stepdaughter and refused specialized treatment, work on his own childhood experiences led him to acknowledge the abuse and to follow through with our referral for further treatment.

Given the special treatment challenges and needs of adult persons who offend, especially those who have done so repeatedly and for long periods, we have chosen to work mostly with juveniles, both children and ado-

---

[1](footnote from page 125) We discuss work exclusively with males who offend, as we do not have experience working with females who offend, and national statistics indicate that sexual abuse is perpetrated overwhelmingly more often by men than by women (Sedlack & Broadhurst, 1996).

lescents. And even in working with juveniles, we further restrict our work to those whose involvement in abusive behavior would be categorized as mild to moderate. Table 7.1 lists risk assessment criteria for juveniles developed by Robert Prentky (1998). As with adults, those juveniles at great risk to reoffend we refer to agencies or practitioners who conduct more specialized treatment. Even with these restrictions, there remains a large group of boys, teens, and young men who have offended and fit into the mild-to-moderate risk categories that we will treat. We hope this chapter will be es-

TABLE 7.1. Juvenile Risk Assessment Scale

High-risk criteria

1. Two or more prior sexual offenses (victims)
2. Clear evidence of predatory behavior
3. Clear evidence of sexual preoccupation
4. Extensive history of impulsive, antisocial behavior
5. Chronic or severe history of substance abuse

Moderate-risk criteria

1. One prior sex offense (victims)
2. Possible or questionable evidence of predatory behavior
3. Possible or questionable evidence of sexual preoccupation
4. Moderate history of impulsive, antisocial behavior
5. Moderate history of substance abuse

Low-risk criteria

1. No prior sex offenses (victims)
2. No clear evidence of predatory behavior
3. No clear evidence of sexual preoccupation
4. Minimal or no history of impulsive, antisocial behavior
5. Minimal or no history of substance abuse

Procedure for classifying risk level

High risk: If three or more are present, or criterion 1 plus any other criteria

Moderate risk: Two criteria from the high-risk group, or any three criteria from moderate risk, or moderate-risk criterion 1 plus any other criteria

Low risk: Low-risk criterion 1 must apply; no high-risk criteria apply; no more than two of the moderate-risk criteria apply (except for criterion 1, which must not apply)

From Prentky (1998). Unpublished scale used with permission of the author. Copyright 1998 by Robert A. Prentky.

pecially useful for other agencies and practitioners who, like ourselves, do not have the expertise to conduct specialized cognitive-behavioral treatment and group programs but are still faced with the need to treat these offending youth and their families.

There are several advantages in focusing on juveniles who offend, especially from a relational approach:

- Because they are younger, they have had less time to develop abusive patterns or to establish pedophiliac[2] tendencies. Research shows that many adult pedophiliacs begin such behavior as teens, a finding that further supports (from a preventive perspective) the need to work with juveniles (Murphy & Smith, 1996).
- Because boys who abuse still live under adult supervision, the initial assessment and ongoing evaluation of progress can include the multiple perspectives provided by boys, family members, teachers, and others, and do not need to rely solely or mostly on self-report of the offending family member, which can be biased in terms of inflating estimates of positive change (Murphy & Smith, 1996).
- Likewise, as opposed to working with an offending adult alone or in groups of others whom he meets only in the treatment setting, when treating an offending juvenile, adult family members can be directly and consistently engaged in the treatment process.

In other words, in contrast to that of adults who offend, the relational context of juveniles is typically more available to assist in promoting treatment goals and monitoring change.

TREATMENT GOALS

The consensus in the literature is that treatment of children and older youths who sexually offend must be abuse-focused (Berliner & Rawlings, 1991). It is also important to address the broader set of psychological and relational concerns that contribute directly or indirectly to the child's offending behavior. Thus, the treatment goals for offending children and teens include the following:

---

[2]Pedophilia is defined as a primary sexual interest in children. Not all child sexual abuse is due to pedophilia.

1. To take 100% responsibility for the abuse and to commit to preventing further abuse.
2. To develop genuine empathy for the abused child and other family members, demonstrated both by repeated statements that evince an authentic shift in perceptions, beliefs, and emotions, and by participating in empathic acts.
3. To address other psychosocial problems (individual and familial) that might facilitate future abuse.

To achieve these goals, the relational approach addresses both the moral and psychological aspects of the abusive behavior in the context of the offending person's family and other significant relationships. We begin by revisiting the issues resulting from treatment being conducted within the larger system of legal action against offending persons.

THE INTERSECTION OF PSYCHOTHERAPY AND SOCIAL CONTROL

Basic Concepts

Therapy with persons who offend is almost always conducted in a context where psychotherapy and social control institutions intersect, each recursively affecting the other. For instance, if helping a young man to take responsibility for the abuse without addressing the legal implications of his doing so, the therapist might not recognize the realistic fears that maintain the youth's denial of his role or the abuse altogether. Likewise, if the therapist focuses solely on legal disincentives for assuming responsibility and does not address the youth's psychological concerns, he or she might overlook the impact of the youth's fears about how his relationship with family members will change.

Guidelines for Practice: Example

An 11-year-old boy insisted, despite a great deal of evidence to the contrary, that he had not molested his 8-year-old stepsister. The therapist spoke to the prosecutor assigned to the case, and he assured us that if the boy received treatment and the parents cooperated in instituting a safety plan, he would not pursue pressing charges. The therapist and parents conveyed this information to the boy and reassured him that acknowledging the abuse would not result in his being "sent away." Despite these reassurances, he continued to deny his abusive behavior.

At this point, the therapist asked him a hypothetical question, one that we often find useful—"Who do you think would be the last person to forgive you if you did this abuse?" Without skipping a beat, he responded, "My mother." This led to a full discussion of how he believed his mother would be enormously disappointed in him. With this relational belief made explicit, the therapist encouraged mother and son to discuss openly the mother's ability to still love him even if he had done something terrible. Only after this reassuring exchange could the boy acknowledge his abusive behavior.

JUSTICE AND CARE: TWO MORAL PERSPECTIVES

Basic Concepts

Although the study of moral development and judgment is itself a complex topic overall, the work of Carol Gilligan and colleagues (Gilligan, Ward, & Taylor with Bardige, 1988) is useful in understanding the moral dilemmas and choices characteristic of the abusive context. Her research distinguishes two fundamental approaches to moral dilemmas and choice. One approach prioritizes concerns about connection, care, and responsiveness to the needs of all involved, while the other privileges concerns about equality and justice. The tendency to make moral decisions within one frame versus another appears gender-related (with girls and women gravitating to care-based, and boys and men gravitating to justice-based, judgments). However, provided that there is attainment of a certain level of cognitive development, many adults of both sexes (as well as older children and teens) have the capacity to solve moral problems through both approaches. Yet as Gilligan notes, children are typically socialized to select one frame over another, and generally, in our society, the justice perspective has subordinated the care perspective. This is so despite research suggesting that empathy develops by the middle of the second year (Walley, 1993). Gilligan suggests that true moral maturity involves the capacity to integrate the two moral "languages" (Gilligan et al., 1988).

In work with boys who offend, the relational approach encourages them to adopt both a justice and a care perspective. From a justice perspective, an essential goal of treatment is that the boy understand that he was 100% responsible for perpetrating the abuse. Boys who have abused often show great difficulty in deeply feeling or at least expressing a grasp of the profound injustice of what they have done (Johnson, 1993). Even when fear of legal reprisals is at a minimum or nonexistent, and even when boys have been reassured by their parent(s) that they will still be loved and not extruded from the family, some boys continue to rationalize, justify, or deny their choice to abuse. In fact, as Johnson notes, "Even being discovered in the act of molesting another child does not necessarily break down the denial of responsibility" (Johnson & Feldmeth, 1993, p. 49).

Guidelines for Practice

Exploring and Expanding Definitions of Self

Exploration of their definitions and accounts of self reveals that many of these boys predominantly view themselves negatively. For example, in a case described earlier, when we asked one 12-year-old boy, who denied having abused his sister, how he would feel about himself if he acknowledged that he had abused her, he answered, "I would completely hate myself." This boy, like others, related a life narrative that was largely empty of pride or self-worth. Even when stories of survival and strength are brought forward, these stories of pride, typically about events in the boy's more distant past, are not ample enough to "stand beside" their more recent acts of betrayal and abuse. To acknowledge to others as well as themselves the extent of the wrongfulness of their acts, and to tolerate the difficult feelings that accompany carefully examining these acts, these boys need others to hold sufficiently positive regard for them to contain the negative self-definitions that would accompany such an acknowledgment. As Walley (1993) writes, "Children who are encouraged to feel good about themselves may be more inclined to empathize with others than children who are preoccupied with personal inadequacies and other concerns about the self" (p. 92). Research has found development of empathy to be associated with positive self-concept (Strayer, 1983), further supporting the importance of helping offending boys to develop positive self-accounts if they are to become empathic with the children they abused.

Thus, treatment of youth who offend often needs to begin by helping them to build a more solid sense of self-worth and pride. Specifically, the therapist stays alert for any talent or particular interest the boy evidences and looks for ways for the boy to show and develop that talent in therapy sessions and share it with family members who can then reflect back positive appraisals that build his sense of pride.

Use of Art Activities to Strengthen Pride in Self

We have found that many of the boys who offended are talented in any number of areas, including art—drawing, clay, graffiti writing. Based on this observation, we worked with an artist (Abbe Steinglass) who created a program for the boys and their mothers that occurred in conjunction with the regular individual and family sessions. Whereas others use art primarily to reveal and work with children's unconscious or otherwise unspoken psychological issues, or to allow symbolic ventilation of pent up feelings (Gil, 1991), we focus almost entirely on praising the artistic activity and production as representative of positive aspects of the self. Although we did not conduct a controlled study on its effectiveness, those boys who received this relational art intervention shared more about the abuse and their responsibility for it than boys treated in the years prior to our starting this intervention. One boy initially said that he knew his abusive behavior was wrong but could not elaborate beyond that. A few weeks after starting the art program and receiving positive comments about his art from the artist, the treatment team, and his mother, he spoke in detail about how he convinced himself that his half-sister really wanted the sexual contact. Another boy, who initially reasoned unempathically that "it was wrong because you could get sent away," experienced positive feedback about his art and only then began to consider how "it is not right to take advantage of someone who is younger and looks up to you."

Talking about Talking and Focusing on the Present

As noted earlier, offending youth are often reluctant to speak about the abuse initially because of fears of legal or other punishment, as well as worries that they will be negatively viewed by the therapist or family members. To focus only on the abuse may result in the boy stating what he imagines the therapist wants to hear. In addition, in a number of cases, the actual abuse has occurred some time earlier, and, as with the abused child, more immediately upsetting may be the events and circumstances following disclosure.

As a result, in order to develop a nonjudgmental treatment relationship and to address the issues most salient to the offending child, therapy typically focuses initially on the most recent events, experiences, or activities in the boy's life. We engage the offending child in Talking about Talking to decide what to discuss in any particular therapy session, when to approach talking about the abuse, how much to talk about it, and when to return to it.

Of course, in commencing work with the abused child, the therapist must tell the offending youth from the outset that the reason for the therapy is that the youth was reported to have been sexually abusive, and the therapist should state the victim's name. The therapist states that at some point, discussion will turn to the abuse but that for the time being the boy can decide what he wants to discuss. If the boy elects to talk about the abuse, the therapist follows his lead. More typically, the boy would rather talk about other things first. These discussions allow him to share his concerns and sources of positive affect and pride, and provide an opportunity for him to describe his experience of important family relationships in a manner less directly influenced by the abuse. Once he becomes comfortable talking about these relationships, it is usually relatively easy for the therapist to guide the conversation into talk about the impact of disclosure on these relationships, then to the impact of the abuse itself, and finally, to an open discussion about the abuse, in which the boy acknowledges (or begins to acknowledge) his responsibility for it.

Example

One teenage boy, who had been removed from his family and placed in residential care, felt confused, frightened, and rejected for having been extruded from his family. In his opinion, his younger stepsister had been seductive. He felt that he was wrong for having her sit on his lap and rub against him but that he didn't deserve to be removed from the home. He believed his stepmother had never liked him and that his father now saw him as bad.

The first part of the therapeutic work with this young man, who came for therapy during his placement in the residential facility, focused on bringing forth his perceptions of his family relationships, both present and past. After a full description, the therapist invited him to consider how the abuse had affected all his relationships. The therapist only moved to the abuse itself after the boy had ample opportunity to reveal and explore a range of thoughts and feelings about the important people in his life. He spoke of anger and pain about his own mother's death and shared his dismay that his stepmother seemed to have little real interest in him. He talked of frustration about his father's strong desire to please his stepmother, even at the expense of protecting his son. And he revealed the painful belief that his father and stepmother preferred their shared biological child to him.

Only after this young man felt heard, understood, and accepted could he allow himself to envision his stepsister's experience and to entertain a different understanding of her behavior toward him. He came to recognize her gestures toward him not as seductive, but as expressing a desire to be accepted by him—a need not so different from his own wishes.

THE SHIFT FROM OTHERS AS OBJECTS TO OTHERS AS SUBJECTS: BUILDING EMPATHY

Basic Concepts

Even when the boys grasp from a justice perspective that what they did was wrong, from a care perspective, they often continue to demonstrate lack of empathy for their specific victim. Until they think about the victimized child as a subject, and not as an object of their sexual or aggressive impulses, these boys are at risk to reoffend. Beyond learning to manage these impulses—a first-order change, albeit a very crucial one—second-order change requires that the boys experience their relational world differently. This shift to seeing themselves as a subject interacting with another subject is at the heart of relationship transformation (Benjamin, 1988).

Of course, many boys who do not sexually abuse girls also objectify them—a practice encouraged by a culture that provides multiple examples of female objectification. However, boys who abuse others often have the additional experience of being themselves objectified through abuse, or of witnessing men engaging in sexual or other violence toward women (Berliner & Elliott, 1996). Although further research is needed to establish more clearly the developmental pathways that heighten the risk of sexual offending (Murphy & Smith, 1996), it is believed that some combination of the broad-based cultural messages regarding male entitlement to sex and the objectification of women, early eroticization, exposure to family violence (sexual and other types), fears of diminished masculinity, low self-esteem, difficulty managing sexual and aggressive impulses, and a fragile attachment to one's caregivers all may contribute to youth engaging in sexually abusive behavior (Gil & Johnson, 1993).

Guidelines for Practice

There are three main practices for working with offending family members to develop empathy for the abused child. Again, although we focus here on children or adolescents who offended, the same practices apply to work with many adults.

1. Deconstructing the abusive acts.
2. Deconstructing a problem situation other than the abuse perpetrated, in which the offending person was hurt or victimized (including instances of his own sexual victimization), and using the

feelings uncovered as a basis for empathy with the child he abused. This practice includes helping the offending member to identify the differences and the similarities between his experience of being victimized or hurt and the empathically imagined experience of the child he abused.

3. Participating in empathic acts such as apology sessions and developing safety plans.

These practices are conducted in a mix of family and individual sessions. As noted earlier, a number of treatment programs for offending youth center on group therapy (Gil & Johnson, 1993; Murphy & Smith, 1996). We have focused on family therapy with individual sessions as needed both because of our general emphasis on working within the child's significant relational context, and because of logistical issues in our treatment center that did not readily permit group therapy.

Often, the offending family member's denial of the facts of the abuse, its impact, or his responsibility for it is supported by similar denial on the part of other family members. As we have emphasized throughout this book, the complex attachments and the loyalty binds that characterize families experiencing relational trauma must be addressed. For instance, if a boy senses that his mother cannot tolerate knowing that he abused a sibling, this will markedly interfere with his ability and willingness to shoulder responsibility and experience empathy. Relational therapy addresses both his internalized premises about himself in relation to others and current interactions with family members that support certain feelings and beliefs over others.

In the therapeutic conversations that occur as the offending person engages in these practices, the two aspects of morality, justice and care, serve as themes that mutually inform one another; that is, as the offending family member increasingly comes to recognize his responsibility for the abuse, he begins to see the abused girl no longer as simply an extension or target of his own needs (an object), but as a person in her own right, with thoughts, desires, and feelings (a subject). This sets the stage for him to imagine how she felt and how his actions violated her desires for herself. And as he becomes increasingly able to empathically imagine her experience of the abuse, he gains a deeper, less abstract sense that what he did was unjust.

We next discuss the details of the first two empathy-building practices (and part of the third—developing a safety plan). The third apology session has several steps and is discussed separately.

Deconstructing the Abuse

Before beginning to deconstruct the abuse, it is critical to clarify the legal status of the boy who abused and the reporting requirements of the therapist. If the family's belief is that it is best not to acknowledge the abuse or the full extent of it because of the potential legal consequences of doing so, this must be addressed fully before deconstructing the abuse. Otherwise, such work will be futile. The therapist should talk with family members about their understanding of the offending child's legal status and also clarify this with larger system professionals (judge, prosecutor, child welfare caseworker) involved with the case. Our experience has frequently been that judges or prosecutors will waive the requirement of therapists to report further confirmation of past incidents of abuse as long as the offending child and family are receiving treatment.

Deconstructing the abusive events involves having the child who abused describe the events slowly, in a step-by-step, "frame-by-frame" manner, and exploring with him the beliefs and assumptions that formed the basis for his actions at each step. We ask him to describe his behaviors and those of the abused child in sequence, as well as memories of his thoughts, feelings, and perceptions at the time (including perceptions of verbal and nonverbal indications of what the abused child might have been feeling). As the beliefs underlying his actions, perceptions, thoughts, and feelings are explored, his accounts of "what happened" often change and expand in ways that allow him to recognize the choices he made and the reasons, however distorted, for these choices. In reciprocal fashion, this then allows for further discussion and questions about his beliefs.

Going over the details of the abuse in this manner can be anxiety provoking for the child. Although some degree of anxiety is certainly appropriate given the behavior being discussed, if the boy feels too overwhelmed, he may shut down or withdraw entirely from therapy. As noted earlier, to avert this, we engage the boy in Talking about Talking—planning the content of the session with him, asking him from time to time if he feels able to proceed or if he would like to talk about something else for a while (e.g., some source of positive feeling or pride), and so on. We usually end such sessions by inviting the boy to comment on the progress he has made toward taking responsibility, encouraging him to feel some pride in coming to terms with a story of shame.

When conducted patiently and nonjudgmentally, deconstructing the abusive events is usually a key practice in assisting the abusing child to take greater responsibility, to grasp better the impact of his behavior, and to identify the sources of his problematic beliefs. Moments in the abuse narrative in which he chose to pursue abuse rather than stop—moments often experienced as fleeting during the actual event—can be slowed down and examined, allowing actions to be linked to the abusing child's underlying premises about himself, girls and sexuality, his family, and so on.

Example

Mike, a 16-year-old teenager with whom we worked, related that during the period of the abuse, he had slept in the same bedroom with his younger sister. On the two occasions when he perpetrated the abuse, Mike had felt sexually aroused in general (not by his sister) and felt he needed to "release" himself. He did so by rubbing his penis between her buttocks while, out of fear, she pretended to be asleep. As we slowed down and deconstructed this sequence and located the beliefs behind his behavior, a much more complex description emerged. The discussion uncovered his beliefs about gender and what it means to be a real man, specific male practices in his family that privileged men's needs over women's, and a concern about his heterosexuality, based on himself having been abused by a man. This fuller description offered many more options for therapeutic intervention. Mike could reflect on the contradiction between the love and respect he had for his mother and some pejorative beliefs about women and their sexuality. He could also reflect on and consider the aspects of his father's attitudes and practices toward women that he wanted to emulate and those he wanted to reject, and this choice could be considered in relationship to the meaning of loyalty toward his father.

Furthermore, as the abuse was unpacked, Mike and the therapist observed that the troubling question about whether Mike was "really a man"—a question that he posed to himself as he compared his own sexual "conquests" to those of his father—seemed to propel him toward "proving" his manhood by seducing girls at school. His abusive acts toward his sister came after days in which he had not been successful in getting a girl's phone number or in having sexual contact. Aroused and frustrated from these unsuccessful pursuits, and chronically aroused from the time of his earlier sexual abuse, he turned for release to his sister.

Having articulated the details of the sequence of beliefs, feelings, and actions leading up to the abuse, Mike and his family could work with the therapist to develop a clear safety plan that prevented Mike from abusing his sister again. Along with this important, practical preventive outcome, the therapy provided Mike an opportunity to articulate and better understand the ideas, feelings, and internal states of arousal that had contributed to his abusive behavior. His initial description of the abuse events was narrow and held few options for change. The fuller, nuanced description that emerged from deconstructing the abuse provided many avenues to explore, to define and redefine, and to suggest intervention in order to prevent further abuse. These are elaborated in Chapter 8, where the case of Mike and his family is described in detail.

Deconstructing an Analogous Experience in Which the Offending Boy Was Hurt or Victimized

Despite attempts to engage them in empathy through deconstructing the abuse they perpetrated, some offending boys continue to express little recognition of the abused girl's experience. Their descriptions are thin, and their major focus remains on their own troubles. With these boys, the therapist can too easily find her- or himself pushing too hard for expressions of empathy, or having blocked, redundant conversations. To counter this unproductive exchange, it is useful to start with a focus on current life situations that trouble the boy and contain material that describes him being mistreated or objectified in some manner. Accepting the boy's initial self-focus avoids a potential struggle to "get him" to become empathic or to focus on the abuse. Free of this struggle, the therapeutic conversation can then focus on deconstructing the boy's own painful experiences and using them as an analogue or bridge to begin to understand what the girl he victimized might have been feeling. Once we identify a link that resonates for him, we articulate it either directly or by asking questions that will help him make a connection between his present experience and the experience of the person he abused. Once he makes the connection, we move to deconstruct the abuse, as described earlier. We then work with him to differentiate his own experiences from those of his victim and help him develop acts of empathy.

Examples

Carl, an 11-year-old boy who participated with his male cousins in abusing Tina, his 8-year-old female cousin, at first denied being a participant. He claimed to have been a reluctant observer. We speculated that because he was severely beaten by Tina's father after disclosure of the abuse, Carl was too fearful of further punishment to acknowledge that he participated in the abuse. After sharing this thought with Carl, as well as telling him he would not be placed out of the home if he acknowledged the abuse (because of his young age and participation in therapy), Carl acknowledged that he did take part in abusing Tina.

Although this was an important step, Carl's lack of empathy for Tina was striking. Instead, he focused on the punishment he received, on how he was pressured into the abuse by his older cousins, and on how he was being ostracized by his extended family. He also focused on how the boy who initiated the abusive behavior and was instrumental in getting Carl to act was not being held more accountable. Initially, we responded to these feelings by exploring what it meant to be one of the guys, what it meant to be accepted, how hard it can be to stand up for one's own beliefs. Although all these themes were worthy of exploration, we remained acutely aware that they centered on Carl and not on the little girl he and his cousins sexually abused. Carl was so preoccupied with the consequences of the abuse for him that there was no room to consider her experience.

Eventually, an event in Carl's life provided us an opportunity to connect his feelings with those of Tina. It occurred during a session in which Carl's father, who had promised to join Carl and his mother in a family session, did not show up. Carl was visibly upset. As it turned out, his father, who had repeatedly let him down, had specifically promised to come to the session. This was very important to Carl, since he felt proud that he was "dealing" with his problems and wanted his father to meet us and hear from us. When asked which word most clearly described how he felt, Carl said, "Betrayed." Quietly, the therapist asked if Carl thought that Tina might have felt the same about him. For the first time, Carl was able to imagine how Tina had counted on him—his affection, his goodwill, his reliability. He even said that as badly as he felt about his father betraying him, his behavior toward Tina was even worse, because he physically harmed her.

In this conversation, Carl moved from a focus entirely on himself to one of empathy for Tina. He could articulate how they shared similar, and different feelings. His mother said that when she had been physically abused by Carl's father, she, too, felt betrayed and violated. The conversation continued and deepened, centering on similarities and differences among Tina's, Carl's, and his mother's experiences.

It then was not a big leap for the therapist to introduce the idea that there are different ways to be a man. Carl, like the young man in the previous example, was invited to consider how he might want to be both like his father and different from him. He also was invited to consider aspects of his mother that he admired and would like to emulate—the idea being that it can be acceptable for boys to aspire to and emulate attributes generally ascribed to women and girls, and that it is often liberating for boys who are constrained by rigid, culturally based definitions of masculinity.

Once the link between Carl's and Tina's experiences was established, we could deconstruct the abuse. Carl described it in detail—what he noticed about Tina's reactions as well as what he now imagined she felt. These sessions were followed by an act of empathy—an apology letter that Carl wrote. The letter reflected the empathy Carl felt for Tina as well as his apology and taking responsibility for what he had done to her.

Sometimes the connecting theme between the offending boy's experience and that of the girl he abused is not immediately evident. In the following vignette, we deconstruct two situations that reveal the feelings, attitudes, and potential of a young man who had demonstrated little empathy for the child he abused. With these characteristics revealed, we could pinpoint what would help him not to behave aggressively in the current situation and develop a bridge to his experiences with abuse both as a victim and as a person who abused another child.

When we met him, Winston had been living for 8 months in a residential facility. He was placed there after abusing his young cousin on one occasion. Winston had lived with his cousin's family after his own mother had left him when he was 4 years old. Though he did not remember it, his aunt reported that he was repeatedly sexually abused when he was 2 years old by an adult relative who was serving time for the abuse. Because Winston's aunt already felt burdened by his presence, she did not think she would be willing to have him return to her home.

Winston was extremely upset about being placed in the residential facility. One reason was that although he was intellectually bright, the limited resources of the facility forced him to attend a special education school. He was also upset that he would never return to his family. By his estimation, the negative impact of the abuse on his life, which seemed now to offer a dismal future, outweighed the seriousness of the single incident of abuse he perpetrated. Although he felt remorseful, he also believed he was being punished too severely for what he did. He reflected on how his cousin was still in the home where he wished to be, and how she had the love and sympathy of the family, which he did not have.

When we first met, Winston was quite despairing. Although we worked with him in the variety of ways described earlier and he did become more available and responsive, we felt he still had not demonstrated enough empathy for his cousin. His narrative and ruminations remained focused on himself and his suffering. Given his circumstances, we understood his fears about his future, his feelings of rejection, and his anger about being with boys who had special needs, and how these could overshadow his feelings of empathy for the girl he abused. Therefore, it seemed important to stay with the concerns and experiences in Winston's present life and be alert for opportunities to use them as analogues and bridges to developing empathy for the cousin he abused.

In the next session, Winston described two incidents from the previous week that seemed to hold possibility for finding an empathic bridge. In one incident, he felt his teacher had mistreated him. Tempted to curse at the teacher and storm out of the room, Winston managed to stay. When we asked him how he decided not to act out, Winston said he reminded himself that this teacher had previously reassured him that he was only in the special education class because the residential facility did not have regular classes. From this comment, Winston felt the teacher recognized that he was academically capable. He felt good about what the teacher said to him. It showed Winston that the teacher regarded him as he wanted to be seen. Winston reflected with us about how he drew on this positive memory of the teacher and, in the moment when he felt provoked, could see the teacher both as unfair toward him in the moment but as previously supportive. By holding both these descriptions, Winston had been able to contain his behavior and not act out.

Another event occurred the same week. This time, Winston looked to the same teacher to intervene on his behalf when another student, Jim, relentlessly pestered him, but to no avail. With his anger mounting, and with no response from the teacher to his requests for intervention, Winston finally flung Jim across the room. Jim lay sprawled out on the floor. When we asked Winston how he felt seeing Jim like this, he said it was funny.

The juxtaposition of these two stories opened several possibilities for therapeutic inquiry. One set of questions focused on Winston's relationship to his teacher. Although in the first event, Winston could hold onto his teacher's positive regard for him and not act out, in the second, Winston described his teacher's lack of response as a failure to protect him.

After arriving at this more complex description of how Winston experienced his teacher's response to him, we turned to a line of questions that focused on the experience of Jim, the boy Winston had hurled across the room. We asked him to describe in detail how Jim was bothering him, what he did, and how Winston reacted each time. We then invited him to speculate on what Jim wanted, why he might have continued despite Winston's rebuffs and warnings. And, again, we asked Winston to use a word that he thought best captured what Jim wanted. When Winston immediately responded that he thought Jim wanted attention, we began to ask about attention in terms of what it means to get attention, what it felt like not to get it, how to try and get it, the ways Winston had gotten attention, the ways he had not, how he felt when he got it, and how he felt when deprived of it. In this exchange, Winston began to see the boy he harmed as wanting some of the same things he wanted. Winston observed how Jim's behavior got worse as he experienced Winston's rejection. As the interaction between the therapist and Winston continued, Winston's narrative about Jim expanded, and he commented that Jim also probably felt unprotected.

We asked Winston if, during the next week, he would begin to observe Jim and, if Jim again behaved in ways that were annoying, to ask him what he wanted. We also suggested that Winston might share with Jim the observation that Jim might want attention from him.

This exercise, which placed Winston in an observing position, provided rich material in the next therapy session. Winston found that by being simultaneously annoyed *and* understanding, he could exercise restraint over his impulses. In both situations, the one with his teacher and this latest experience with Jim, a more complex understanding of the other person enabled Winston to behave differently. The therapist and Winston then explored how Winston could help Jim behave in less annoying ways.

In subsequent sessions, Winston described how he had tried to imagine someone's experience before acting on whatever he himself might have been feeling. For instance, when he was shoved in the lunch line by another boy who was horsing around, Winston took a moment to realize the boy had not meant to insult him or start a fight, and so Winston did not shove back. When he once missed the bus back to the residence on Sunday and was penalized for it, he could imagine the concern of the cottage staff for him and for making sure that rules were followed rather than just simmering in his own irritation and anger about the restrictions placed on him.

These therapeutic conversations revealed that when Winston could hold more than one description of both himself and the other person with whom he was interacting, he could practice restraint. Furthermore, when Winston could reflect on the motivations of the other person, he could begin to identify with that person's needs. This more empathic understanding could be extended to his abusive behavior with his younger cousin. When the therapist asked him to connect his observations about his experience with his horseplaying classmate to his interaction with his cousin, he quickly related how he could see her as both annoying and wanting his attention. In the past, he had only experienced her as relentlessly teasing him. Considering her more benign motivation (one that he could identify with), while at the same time recognizing how its expression greatly annoyed him, Winston could begin to imagine her experience of the abuse without feeling that it negated his feelings. The both–and thinking allowed him to see her as feeling frightened and harmed by the big cousin she looked up to and expected to protect her.

With these new insights, Winston could add far more emotional and physical detail to his description of the abuse. He then asked the therapist if she thought his cousin would remember what happened when she got older. The therapist responded that she might or might not recall the abuse in her mind, but she might react negatively to being touched, without knowing why—almost like the body remembered what the mind could not. She then suggested that perhaps his body remembered the abuse inflicted on him when he was 2 years old, even though he could not recall it in his mind. She asked Winston to imagine how a 2-year-old boy might have felt. Through this hypothetical conversation, Winston came to appreciate the fear, confusion, anger, and pain he must have experienced. The therapist then suggested that maybe when he was shoved, or pestered, or felt he was treated badly, he could feel it in his body like he did when he was 2 years old. However, when he was 2, he was helpless; now, he could protect himself. Ironically and unfortunately, on some occasions, he used a way of protecting himself that hurt or abused someone else. The therapist suggested that, together, they would continue to explore ways he could protect himself without harming others.

Sometimes, therapists are concerned that if a boy who abused was himself abused, discussing his own experience could too easily become an excuse for his behavior. We believe this only happens if discussing the boy's own abuse is viewed as sufficient treatment, rather than using it as a step to create an emotional and cognitive basis for empathy into the experience of the child he abused. As an example, we encountered a teenage boy who had been incarcerated for months and had received abuse counseling in a correction facility. Though he was abused by an older relative on repeated occasions, the entire focus of treatment was on what he had perpetrated. The following dialogue is included to illustrate the potential of including both discourses in one session. It is also a good example of use of Talking about Talking and the Decision Dialogue.

THERAPIST: We were talking last time, and both of us were trying to understand what you did to your sister and about the abuse that your cousin did to you. And we discussed how in your previous therapy you only talked about the abuse you had done to your sister and not at all about your experience of being abused.

JACK: Right.

THERAPIST: Well, I think we began to think about whether or not you wanted to discuss what happened to you.

JACK: Yeah. I was thinking that it might help to talk about it, though I am not sure it will help me.

THERAPIST: OK, I think that you are raising a good question, so perhaps we should talk about talking about it.

JACK: Well, I think it would help to talk about it to stop the secrecy stuff. Also, maybe I will remember more. If I can tell someone about it and take it slowly, maybe more and more will come up.

THERAPIST: You can decide how much to talk about. You can be in charge and say when we have talked enough about it. Do you think you can be that direct with me?

JACK: (*Smiles*.) I don't know, I'm not used to it, but I will try.

THERAPIST: OK. I will try to help by asking you if we have talked enough, or whether we should talk about other things for awhile. So, together, we'll be paying close attention to how you are feeling about remembering.

Dialogue from the next session:

THERAPIST: OK. Since life is good in the present and was problematic in the past, is it all right if we spend some time talking about a time when it was hard?

JACK: Sure.

THERAPIST: Is it really OK, or are you being polite?

JACK: No. I don't mind going back. I am looking more forward to good times in the future, but like we decided, it will be better to no longer have this shameful secret.

THERAPIST: I am all for future good times for you.

Jack then begins to describe his memory of being abused. It is primarily a visual memory. He describes it and the therapist asks if he remembers how he felt. He responds by saying how he is angry with his cousin. The cousin is someone Jack looked up to, someone whose affection he wanted, someone he wanted to please. Jack spontaneously reflects that about his own abuse he is really angry, and yet this is just what he did to his sister. He says, "It [the feelings] always backfires. I want to kill him and then I think that I did the same thing to my sister—I took advantage of her—and then I hate myself."

As the conversation continues, Jack describes how he imagines his sister felt, and the therapist asks him if he has ever talked with her about it; he says no. The therapist asks him if he thinks it would be useful to have this conversation with her. When he says yes, the therapist asks him what he would like to talk about with her. Jack responds with several ideas. He wants to know if she is angry with him. He wants her to know that he, too, was abused, and that he might know how she felt. He wants her to know that he knows how wrong it was. He wants to know what it was like for her. He wants to know if she is now alright. As he elaborates these themes and thinks of other topics, he observes that if they were to begin to speak together, it would probably allow them to open up a lot of conversation at home. Jack says, "I could probably go up to her and ask how she is feeling and she wouldn't see me as such a threat. I would be more comfortable talking to her."

As can be seen from this example, when a boy's own abuse is explored both to help him heal from it and to help him locate feelings that allow him to empathize with his victim, he does not view his own abuse as an excuse. Quite the contrary, coming to terms with it deepens the sense of responsibility he has for having perpetrated an act that was painful for himself when he was the victim. The therapist must extend the conversation to include the differences as well as the similarities between the two experiences. These distinctions ensure that the person who abused clearly sees the other as a person with her own subjective experience.

AN ACT OF EMPATHY AND RESPONSIBILITY: THE SAFETY PLAN

Basic Concepts

No matter what the nature, level of severity, and duration of the abuse to date, it is important to clarify with both offending and nonoffending family members that there is no "cure" for sexual offending (Murphy & Smith, 1996) and that there is always the possibility that the offending family member may again abuse. Current studies suggest that the recidivism rate for persons who offend after completing outpatient treatment programs is anywhere between 0% and 17%, as compared to 1% to 42.9% for untreated offending family members (Murphy & Smith, 1996). However, as Murphy and Smith point out, the lower recidivism rates for those treated may have as much or more to do with the fact that those in treatment are more closely monitored during and after treatment (in aftercare programs) than those not in treatment, rather than resulting from the effectiveness of the treatment per se.

Guidelines for Practice

In the relational approach, there are several points at which a safety plan is enacted. Prior to beginning treatment, the therapist needs to establish where the offending family member is living. If he is not in prison, residential treatment, or some other supervised setting, it must be clearly established with social service and legal professionals involved in the case who will be responsible for monitoring the behavior of the offending person and the safety of the abused child. The therapist must be clear with everyone involved that he or she cannot assume this monitoring function. If CPS or the courts have approved the offending person living in the home, contingent on his receiving treatment, the therapist needs to be clear with these larger systems and with the family about requirements for written or other reports.

Once the treatment begins, if the offending person is living in the home or has access to the abused child, this needs to be addressed in a first session, and a safety plan developed. Given that the offending family member may not have much empathy and may not yet have taken 100% responsibility for the abuse, it may not be possible to include him in safety planning at the beginning of treatment. Safety planning at this stage needs to done by the adult, nonoffending family members and others in a position to safeguard the child.

However, once the offending member takes responsibility for the abuse and shows signs of genuine empathy, he can participate in developing, implementing, and monitoring the plan—always under the supervision of a nonoffending parent who can truly protect the abused child. By viewing participation in safety planning as a concrete, action-oriented extension of the new feelings and beliefs he has about what he did, the offending family member deepens his commitment to responsibility and empathy. There is an excellent example of safety planning, as well as the next topic, the apology session, in Chapter 8, in the discussion of therapy with Mike and his family.

THE APOLOGY SESSION

Basic Concepts

Participating in an apology session is one of the most powerful acts of responsibility and empathy an offending family member can do. A number of authors (Madanes, 1990: Trepper & Barrett, 1989) have described formats for apology sessions. Ours incorporates some of the points made by these authors. As always, we are interested not in guiding families through a preset script, but in setting up the possibility for them to create their own, unique experience.

Guidelines for Practice

• *Step 1: Work with the offending family member individually to ensure that he takes 100% responsibility.* Obviously, the first step is to ensure that the offending family member no longer views anyone but himself as responsible for the abuse. He must also be truly remorseful, demonstrate a grasp of the emotional impact of his behavior, and have empathy for the abused child and other family members whom he hurt through his behavior.

• *Step 2: Work with the offending family member to refine his apology and sense of full responsibility.* The therapist needs to talk with the offending person about what he wants to say in his apology, to whom, and how he wants to phrase it. As the offending family member tries out some sample phrases, the therapist may note either that the offending person really seems to understand his responsibility for the abuse, or he still has some lingering confusion about this. For instance, if the offending family member says something to the effect of, "I'm really sorry for how I hurt you. I guess I just lost control because of my drinking" or "I'm sorry for what I did. I guess I didn't listen when you told me to stop," he will need help to see that in a subtle way, he still does not take 100% responsibility for the abuse. For instance, in the first sample phrase, the offending family member seems to blame his drinking, while in the second, he implies that the child was still responsible for telling him to stop (and he just failed to listen). Working on the phraseology of an apology can therefore give the offending family member an opportunity to refine his understanding of his responsibility for the abuse.

One point that is important to emphasize with the offending family member is that his apology must be "freely given"; that is, he should not feel coerced to apologize, and most importantly, *he should not expect forgiveness from the abused child*. The child must be free to accept or reject the apology, to say something or say nothing. Otherwise, she may feel guilty for not forgiving him, adding to what may already be a high degree of self-blame.

• *Step 3: Make sure that the nonoffending parent views the offending family member as 100% responsible.* Before bringing the offending family member, nonoffending parent, abused child, siblings, and other relevant family members together for an apology session, the therapist needs to make sure that the nonoffending parent and other adult family members involved have also come to an understanding that the victimized child was not responsible for the abuse. Prior to the apology session, the nonoffending parent may still blame herself somewhat for the abuse. The formal apology by the offending family member may help to end this self-blame, so it is not necessary for the nonoffending parent to have stopped blaming herself prior to the session. But it is critical that the nonoffending parent clearly support the child and view her as innocent prior to the offending family member's apology. Otherwise, a situation might occur in therapy, especially when the offending family member is a juvenile, in which the offending family member apologizes and the nonoffending parent defends him in front of the abused child.

• *Step 4: Establish that the abused child wants an apology session.* It is, of course, important to work with the abused child and nonoffending parent to talk about what an apology session might be like, to find out if the child wants one, and if so, to explore what she would want to hear. It is also important to let the child know that she will not be asked to forgive the offending family member—that she should not feel pressured to do so. With every family we've seen, when an apology has been possible (when the offending person has been involved or reachable by letter), the child has welcomed the opportunity.

• *Step 5: The sequence of the apology session.* Once the preparatory work of Steps 1–4 has been completed the therapist arranges with the family to hold the apology session. She or he begins the session with an outline of what will happen—something to the effect of, "So, we're meeting together today because your father/brother/uncle/cousin wanted to apologize to you about the abuse." The therapist reminds everyone that this will be an apology that requires no response from the child or anyone else in the family—especially that the child will not be required to accept the apology or offer forgiveness, and that the offending family member should not ask for forgiveness.

The offending family member is then asked to say what he wants to say, and other members are invited to say what they want to say. Although the focus of an apology session should be on the abused child, if the family spontaneously expresses pride in the offending family member for his statements, the therapist can support this and then ask them to state their pride in the abused child in terms of how she has handled the abuse experience, the therapy, and so on.

When the apology and immediate reactions have ended, the therapist asks the child if she would now like to meet individually or with other family members to discuss her feelings about the apology. The key is that the child is put in charge of this process, without pressuring her to make a decision.

Following an apology session, family members are likely to experience a wide range of thoughts and feelings. All members should be given an opportunity to discuss their feelings and thoughts, and comment on how they believe this session will affect each other and the family's healing from the incest experience. These follow-up discussions can occur immediately after the apology as already described, or later, in family or individual sessions.

Variations: Apology by Letter

When the offending family member is incarcerated or otherwise not available for an apology session (e.g., when he is out of the country), he can still offer a formal apology by letter that can be used in an individual session with the child and/or in a family session with whomever else is available. The procedure is essentially the same as described earlier, although the therapist goes through Steps 3 and 4 prior to contacting the offending family member. Once the child seems ready to hear an apology, and the nonoffending parent agrees to the importance of the child hearing directly from the offending family member that he takes 100% responsibility, the therapist contacts the offending family member by letter. The therapist informs him of the purpose of the apology, and, as best as can be done by letter, encourages him to go through Steps 1 and 2. The offending family member then sends the apology letter to the therapist, who screens it and makes sure it does not need to be refined further (Step 2) before being presented to the child. The letter is also discussed with the nonoffending family member to get her thoughts on whether it is ready to be read to or by the child.

Once fully approved, the letter is read to the child or by her in an individual or family session, whichever she prefers. The letter is then discussed in a manner similar to the discussion of the offending person's verbal apology. An example of an apology by letter is presented in Case 2 in Chapter 8.

SUMMARY

In this chapter, we described applying the principles and practices of the re-lational approach to work with the offending family member, especially ju-venile offending members. Relational treatment is most appropriate for children and teenagers who offended, and for those whose pattern of of-fending would be categorized as mild to moderate in severity. Adults and more severely-offending youth are referred for other treatments, sometimes after an initial phase of relational treatment. The goals of treatment in-clude the offending family member taking 100% responsibility for the abuse; development of genuine empathy for the abused child and other family members; and addressing of other psychological and behavioral is-sues that may put the offending person at risk of re-abusing. Many of the therapeutic practices that achieve these goals are the same as those used in work with the abused child: expanding positive self accounts through both–and thinking and amplifying stories of pride; and use of Talking about Talking and the Decision Dialogue to give the abusing child a sense of safety and control in the process of therapy, as well as to help him build a sense of responsibility and appropriate agency. In addition, work with the offending member involves practices that build empathy, especially de-constructing the abuse he perpetrated and discussing experiences in which he was hurt or even abused. Finally, the offending family member is in-volved in apology sessions with the abused child other family members, and in planning for the continued safety of the abused child, and in a sense, his own safety.

We turn now to three extended case descriptions that further explicate the details of the relational approach to treatment of incest.

Chapter Eight

Three Cases

In this chapter, we present three extended accounts of families in treatment to illustrate the theoretical and practical points described in earlier chapters. Our hope is that the reader will obtain from these a clear, detailed sense of how the relational approach works. For each case, we begin by introducing the issues highlighted, present sections of the treatment in chronological sequence, intersperse remarks that highlight dilemmas and choice points, and link the case to the broader ideas and techniques of the relational approach that help to negotiate these dilemmas. Although each case was chosen to highlight certain key issues, we have included enough detail about the entire treatment to allow each case to stand alone.

CASE 1: ORGANIZING AND SEQUENCING THE TREATMENT—CO-CREATING THE THERAPEUTIC SYSTEM

It is always important, and sometimes critical, to think carefully about how to organize the treatment. When the therapy is not going well, we often ask

151

ourselves if we have overlooked important relationships that now constrain the persons in treatment. We regularly consider two questions: "Do we have the right people in the room?", and in our conversations with the family members present, "Are there family members to whom we have not paid attention who might be influencing the ability of others in the room to experience feelings, share opinions, remember events, and express themselves?" More than once, we have discovered that important missing family members create loyalty binds for the child who has been abused, or for the nonabusing, or abusing, parent.

For example, a mother of an abused child wanted to prosecute her husband, the child's stepfather. Yet each time she decided to do it, she changed her mind. It took some time until we learned that her mother-in-law, who was like a mother to her, implored her not to press charges against her son. Her mother-in-law made it clear that if she were to decide to do it, she would not only lose her husband but also his mother. Only after this became clear could we address the loyalty bind that created an intense, paralyzing enactment of this woman's ambivalence.

Powerful loyalty binds may exist even when the person is not directly or regularly involved in the family's life, is not living with or near the family, or even is dead. In these instances, it is important to bring forth the beliefs family members hold about absent parents, grandparents, siblings, and other important persons. A question helps bring forth these relationship descriptions: "Is there anyone who doesn't know about what has happened, who would have some strong feelings about it?"

In addition to neglecting important persons in the family's life, therapy may not proceed well because important steps have been skipped in the sequence. For instance, we usually find we cannot engage the mother or child to talk about the abuse before they have a chance to talk about how the disclosure of abuse was handled by the wider system (i.e., the investigative procedure, the medical exam, other contact with social services). If the child underwent many interviews with police, CPS, law guardians, or physicians, the family's experience of these interviews must be addressed before moving to the abuse itself. If not, the mother may seem guarded, and the child will often seem uncooperative, noncommunicative, or badly behaved.

The following case well illustrates the importance of thinking carefully about who needs to be invited into the "therapeutic system," when and how they are invited, as well as the importance of engaging families to collaborate with the therapist in directing the sequence of topics discussed and treatment modalities used.

The Initial Phone Call

One afternoon, I[1] received a call from an elderly Italian American woman named Daisy, who said she wanted help for her family. She was a nurse and had been shown a film on incest and its deleterious effect over generations. Daisy said that once she realized that abuse could be repeated by the next generation if not treated, she had gone to visit her sister Linda, who agreed for the family to obtain help for both Linda's 10-year-old granddaughter, Sandra—the child who had been abused—and Linda's grandson Mike, who had abused Sandra. Daisy and Linda also knew that Mike had been abused by a neighbor when he was 6 years old. When I asked Daisy to describe the situation, she said that Sandra had disclosed to her mother, Betty (Linda's daughter-in-law), 4 years earlier and that Betty had confided in both Daisy and Linda, who was raising Mike. (Mike's mother died when he was 1 year old.) Linda responded by speaking to Mike, now age 16, who promised never to touch Sandra again. Betty also asked Sandra regularly if Mike was "bothering her," and she said he was not. During this initial call, I asked who else in the family knew about the abuse. Daisy said that the only person in the immediate family who did not know was James, Mike and Sandra's father (who was also Linda's son, Betty's husband, and Daisy's nephew). She said he could not be told what had occurred and sounded anxious even at the thought of his finding out. When I asked why, without hesitating, she said, "Because he would kill Mike if he knew." I asked if she meant this literally, and she said, "Absolutely." When I asked who else agreed with this, Daisy answered that the rest of the family agreed.

I told Daisy that I thought the situation with James, the children's father, required a more lengthy conversation and suggested that the family and I continue to discuss it in person. I then asked Daisy who she thought should be involved. Daisy suggested herself, her sister Linda, and Sandra's mother, Betty. Daisy then asked if we would see Sandra also, and I said I thought it best to figure out first how to handle their concern about the father knowing. I said I knew they were eager to help Sandra, but in our experience, it is important first to figure out and agree on who needs to be involved in that process. I also said that I would have to call the CPS and ascertain the legal requirements given that the abuse had taken place 4 years earlier and had not been reported.

---

[1]Marcia Sheinberg was the therapist.

Discussion

The family believed that to include the father of both the child who was abused and the child who abused was dangerous. Because this was the extent of information I had at this time, I did not insist that Sandra and Mike's father be asked to participate in the first meeting. However, I thought it best not to see the children until this matter was resolved. The attention we give to organizing a case reflects our strong belief that therapy will not go well if we rush the process, regardless of how compelling the desire to help a child who has been abused. We remain mindful that if not sensitively introduced to the child, with the support of the family, therapy has the capacity to worsen trauma.

The First Session

The three women came to the initial meeting that very week and reiterated much of what Daisy had communicated on the phone. Betty added that she particularly wanted help for Sandra now, because Sandra had been saying that she did not like how she looked, and Betty felt this negative self-image might be because of the earlier abuse. All three women were convinced that there had not been any further incidents, since Sandra was open with them, and her mother had asked her directly. They also said she had not evidenced any symptoms.

The women spoke of how Mike was very close to Betty and Daisy, as well as to Linda, whom he considered his mother. The women were also very close. In fact, the proximity of the two families was such that they often saw one another on a daily basis. And though James came to Linda's home most evenings to play checkers with her, all three women agreed that since James had a bad temper, it was best not to share too much with him. I asked questions about the extent of his temper-driven behavior, including: "Has he ever hit any of you? Has he hit the children? Has he gotten into fights at work or in the neighborhood? Does he drink or use drugs that might influence his behavior?" The answers were all negative. What he did do, according to the women, was get angry and yell or get bossy. They felt, however, that he would definitely reject Mike if he knew what had happened. I asked them, if Mike were present, what would he say? Linda was quick to respond: Mike worried that his father would not allow him to stay in the family. And they did not see the point of telling James, when all they wanted was for us to talk with Sandra and Mike, so they could be sure that both kids would be OK.

Although I was respectful of the family's resolution to keep "family business" from James, I also wondered how it might be for Sandra to feel that she could not say anything about the therapy to her father. I said I was concerned that it might make her feel that she had done something so wrong that it had to be kept a secret. I also took the opportunity to speak about other children I had worked with who did not tell about the abuse because they thought they were bad, and how hard we worked with these girls in order for them to become certain that it was not their fault. Though Sandra had told her mother about the abuse and had not kept it a secret, Betty said she could see how Sandra could get mixed up about the reason for keeping the therapy a secret from her father. However, she was concerned about Mike and also wanted to protect him from his father's wrath. I also shared with them the position taken by CPS: that because the family had actively sought treatment for both children, and because the abuse had occurred 4 years ago, it would only need to be reported for investigation if further incidents were revealed in therapy. After hearing this, the family decided to continue in treatment and include James.

Discussion

The dilemma at this point centered on how to maintain a collaborative stance with the family even when their ideas about how to proceed with treatment differed greatly from our own. Although the women wanted me to see the children alone, and without informing their father, I felt this could compromise their comfort in therapy, decrease its effectiveness (for all the reasons we have discussed about the benefits of the relational approach), and ultimately might create more problems for them with James if/when he found out. The challenge here for the collaboratively minded therapist is always to consider respectfully the ideas and wishes of the family, while feeling free to disagree respectfully and offer a different perspective—even to insist respectfully on a certain approach based on the therapist's own experience and clinical judgment. In our thinking, true collaboration of all sorts recognizes that different people bring different types of experiences and expertise to the act of problem solving, as well as different limits on what they are willing to do or not do in a situation. As therapists, the key to avoiding a hierarchical position with families is to be transparent about our positions and decisions, explaining them clearly and openly. Family members then have the information they need to understand our rationale and to decide whether they can work with it or wish to seek counsel elsewhere.

So, although I felt my expertise as a therapist warranted standing by the idea of waiting to see Sandra until her father had been informed, I viewed the women as the experts on the personal qualities of their family members, and so took seriously the family's fear that James could harm Mike. Though it seemed that a circular description might explain an aspect of James's temper—in that the more James is left out of the loop, the more he shows his temper, and the more intimidating his temper, the more he is left out, I chose not to challenge the women to think differently about his behavior at that time, especially because I did not want to question their sense that he could reject Mike. Rather, I went with the description offered by the women who knew him.

Telling James

I asked if we could think together about how they could sequence what they told James about the abuse in a manner least likely to arouse his ire. After more discussion about what to say first, next, and so on, we talked together about who should tell him, and even where he should be told. The three women agreed that Linda should tell him. They explained that, as she was James's mother, he respected her the most. They said that Daisy, though she understood the most about abuse, was not as close to James, and that because his wife Betty was quite a bit younger than he, James did not respect her much. They thought that Linda should tell him when they were alone at her house. They also decided that Linda would first tell James about Mike's own abuse, then tell him about Mike's abuse of Sandra.

Discussion

Based on the women's reporting that despite his temper, James had never actually been physically violent (or even physically threatening), and Mike's sense that he would not be physically hurt by his father, I felt safe suggesting a possible way to begin to include the children's father in the treatment. Once again, in our approach to collaboration, we feel comfortable making suggestions we think might be helpful, but we do so in a manner that makes clear that the suggestions are open for comment, further inquiry, and dismissal. In other words, we try not to "fall in love" with our ideas but do offer what we think might be useful.

In this instance, the family members considered my suggestion of starting treatment with Sandra only after her father was told about the abuse, but again asked about my conducting therapy according to their idea that James not be included or told about it. Because I felt it would be destructive to have Sandra keep it a secret, I could not abide by their plan. I had to be willing to lose the family. We do not view a disagreement of this nature as a power struggle but, rather, as a natural process in which the opinions of both the therapist and family members are openly discussed and respected. In this context of mutual respect, each person can hear the perspective of the others and make decisions.

James joined the women for the next session, and I asked that we include Peter,[2] who would work with Mike. The session focused on James's reaction to the abuse, and what became apparent was that he was primarily upset about having not been informed. He kept saying that he just could not understand why he had not been told for 4 years. The women were quiet and I asked if I might share my understanding. With their agreement, I suggested that I thought the women were protecting James and Mike's relationship. James seemed interested in this idea and asked what I meant. I said that it seemed to me that they did not want to do anything that would risk his rejecting Mike. He said he would not reject Mike. At this point, I said that I believed James could really help both his children. Peter added that he felt that helping both children required all of us, and Betty said, "Like a team."

The remainder of the session focused on how we would all work. It was decided that Peter would spend time with Mike individually, as well as with Mike and James together, and that I would work with Sandra. Both of us would be present for full family sessions. Everyone thought that for my first session with Sandra, only Betty (her mother) should also be present. Otherwise, there would be too many adults, which might be intimidating for Sandra.

Discussion

We think that, when appropriate, it is important to identify honorable intentions behind some actions that on the surface seem deceitful or are hurtful. (We never frame abusive behavior in this way, as there are no honestly honorable intentions behind such behavior.) If we had responded to James's upset with anything that suggested his bad temper was the reason he was not told, he would probably have become defensive. To suggest that the women did not tell him so as to preserve his relationship with his son allowed him to move beyond his anger at being left out. In this accurate, al-

---

[2]Peter Fraenkel

beit partial description of events, he is neither blamed or shamed, and the women's actions can be viewed not as a manifestation of a coalition against him, but as an attempt to prevent rupture of one of his most important family relationships. Although James's reactivity did become a focus later in the treatment—both in his relationship with his son and his wife—it did not make sense to confront him about it in this first session. In fact, it was addressed indirectly in that the women noted their fear that he would become so angry at Mike that he would reject him.

Regarding the decision that I work with Sandra and Peter work with Mike, although in this case the therapist–client relationships ended up being same-sex pairs, the gender match was not deliberate and is usually not something we do unless the family requests it. In this case, I had already developed a relationship with the women, so continuing with Sandra seemed to be a natural extension of the work so far.

Working with the Abused Child: Talking about Talking

One week later, I met with Sandra and her mother. Sandra was shy with me and a little apprehensive. After asking her a few questions about herself, I suggested she use the chalkboard and tell a story about a little girl. Sandra seemed to relax as she drew and told quite an elaborate story. As she developed her plot, I asked some questions, to which she responded, and in a short time, the flow between us seemed quite easy. After she finished the story, I asked if she thought we talked enough for today or if there were some more things she might want to talk about. She answered that we had talked enough. I then asked if she felt like we were getting to know each other a little bit. She said yes, and I asked if there was anything she wanted to know about me. She wanted to know whether I had any children. After I answered her, I asked if it was OK for me to tell her about what I do with the children and families that come to the clinic. She said yes, and I told her that I meet and work with families like her family, where little girls like herself have had experiences in which they've been taken advantage of sexually. I said they come here and talk and play. They talk about themselves and their feelings about themselves and what happened to them. And if they have questions, they ask. I said that sometimes they like to talk alone, without their mothers there, and sometimes they talk with their mothers, too, and that they are the ones to decide. I then asked Sandra if she wanted to spend any time alone with me that day, or if she preferred to wait. Nodding to Betty, I added that her mother had said it was OK for her to meet with me alone (Betty nodded); Sandra looked at her mother, who said that it was OK. Then Sandra answered, "Today."

Discussion

The message we try to give all family members is that the abuse is not the only aspect about them that interests us. At the same time, we note that we will pay particular attention to the abuse. We believe it is crucial in the first session to state clearly the purpose of the treatment so that the child is not left in suspense and is given permission and a first actual opportunity to determine when and how much we will talk about the abuse. So with Sandra, I began telling a story to connect with her, so as to avoid asking her a series of questions for which she did not seem ready. Telling a story is fun, it is not directly about the child, and it gives therapist and child something to which they can mutually relate. In contrast to a more classical psychodynamic approach, where the focus on stories in therapy is on the unconscious meaning, including the transference, we view the telling of stories and related imaginative productions—role plays, dreams, fantasies—as flexible tools to use in a variety of ways, depending on the needs of the therapy at the moment. Sometimes we focus on the content of stories, although not on what they reveal about intrapsychic conflict, or even so much what they show about the child's transference to the therapist, but, rather, on what they reveal about the child's understanding and concerns about her current family relationships (see the case of Laurie in Chapter 2). At other times, as we did in the current case, we use story creation as a modality through which to connect in a manner that is experienced as less threatening by the child and even fun. Stories, drawings, and play in general also provide a resource of activities from which we can draw when the child wants to take a break from talking about the abuse and related topics. Although we do not use the notion of transference in our work (because our focus is on strengthening the child's relationships with actual family members, rather than working on these indirectly through examining her relationship with us), we certainly are always attuned to the child's feelings about us, and invite open discussion of these feelings in language appropriate to the developmental stage of the child.

In this particular session, although her mother was in the room during the storytelling, I spoke more with Sandra and did not invite Betty into the conversation as much as I might have had I not already spent so much time with her. Furthermore, given that I had delayed seeing Sandra for a few weeks in order to set up the therapy, I now wanted to honor Betty's urgent wish that I begin work with Sandra. Once Sandra's story seemed complete, I chose to be explicit about the purpose of their coming to therapy. Before telling Sandra, I asked if she wanted to know what I do—again, to involve her as much as possible in decisions about what she talked about in therapy, rather than my just launching into a description. I did not ask her to say why she thought she was here—first, because I knew from her mother that she knew, but also because this question can put the child on the spot, forcing her to talk about the abuse (even by simply naming it to explain why she is here). Instead, I named it, stating clearly that I work with children who have been abused. I phrased it in this way to let her know that she was not the only little girl to whom something like this has happened, and that, while we can have fun together, we can also be serious and talk about painful, frightening things.

Sandra was extremely lively when she and I met alone. I asked about her little brother and she told me how grown up he tried to act. She imitated him so well that both of us were laughing. She also talked about other family members, including Mike. She described how he would say to her, "Honey, do you love me?" She said that when she then said, "No," he'd laugh and say, "Yes, you do." She then said that when she and her mother were in the waiting room, they talked about Mike, and her mother asked if she was afraid of him. She answered that she was afraid. I asked her why and she said, "Cause I'm scared that he might do it again."

Discussion

At this point in the conversation, Sandra herself introduced the topic of the abuse. We find that children will initiate talking about the abuse when the context feels safe, when they believe that they can talk about many aspects of their lives (not only the abuse), and when they can say yes or no to what is talked about.

Sandra began to cry. I asked her if she would tell me what Mike did to her. She continued crying, and I asked if she would like me to hold her hand. She nodded yes, and we held hands for awhile. She then looked at me and said, "I will tell you."

Discussion

Sandra had clearly decided to speak about the abuse. My offer to hold her hand and to wait for her to decide to talk to me about the abuse gave her the room to decide for herself. The abuse was her experience, and I could be her witness but I was also quite willing to end the session with her not telling me about it. In this way, the child exercises control over the telling, which promotes her sense of personal agency.

Sandra went on to describe in explicit detail what Mike did to her. She reported that the abuse occurred on two occasions. My comments were limited to questions that clarified aspects of the events. Tearfully, almost in a whisper, she described all she could remember. I then suggested that when we met next time, we could talk more about her feelings about it, her questions, or whatever she liked. Before we ended the session, I returned to her initial statement about being afraid of Mike and suggested that we talk this over with her mother. I asked if she would like for her mother to make sure that she was never left alone with Mike. She immediately said yes, and I asked if she wanted me to tell her mother alone or with her present. She said we could be together, but I should say it.

Discussion

The material from the child's individual session that was brought into a family session (with mother and daughter) related to the family protecting her. In keeping with our principle of maintaining a client-determined agenda, the material for the mother–daughter session is specified by the immediate need of the child rather than by a preset agenda on the part of the therapist. Through the Decision Dialogue, the child is made a full participant in deciding what to bring to the conjoint session, as well as how her concerns should be communicated. If a child does not want to discuss her concerns with her mother, I focus on her reasons for this and, in this way, learn more about the child's perception of herself and her relationships with other family members, rather than immediately insisting that we need to tell her mother. In other words, if in the Decision Dialogue we learn that the child does not wish to bring back her concerns to the family, we switch to Talking about Talking and, through this process, gain a better understanding of the beliefs and premises that influence her unwillingness to turn to family members. With these concerns expressed, we can then decide with the child how best to address her concerns with the family.

As I left to get Betty, Sandra selected a puzzle and immediately began to work on it. Her resilience was apparent as she went from a very upsetting description of the abuse she'd endured to actively engaging in play. When her mother and I returned, she was lying on the floor, working on this elaborate puzzle. Upon seeing her daughter so engaged, Betty commented that Sandra loved puzzles. I said to Betty that I thought she had done a terrific job raising her daughter. She thanked me, and I said that she must be very proud of herself. She smiled and said she was. After a little more of this dialogue, I said that one concern emerged from my meeting with Sandra: that she was scared of being with Mike, afraid that he could "do it" again, and that she did not feel safe. Betty nodded in apparent understanding. I went on to say that, if Betty agreed, I thought Sandra should never be left alone with him. Betty immediately said that she could make sure of that. At this point, Betty asked her daughter if it was okay to be with Mike when the family was all around or did she not want to be with him at all. Sandra said it was OK as long as she was never left with him alone. Betty said she would talk to everyone else in the family as well to ensure that it never happened. She also said she would talk directly to Mike and tell him that he would no longer be allowed to be alone with Sandra. Betty again asked her daughter if it this plan was OK and Sandra, smiling and visibly relieved, said yes.

Discussion

In this brief meeting, Sandra actively participated in deciding what would make her feel secure, and her mother was given the opportunity to demonstrate to her daughter that she would listen and take seriously her concerns. The need to protect Sandra both emotionally and physically was not didactically delivered to the mother by a therapist. To deliver this suggestion as a lecture or advice runs the risk of patronizing the parent. Rather, the process of conversation itself created the context in which the child's issues emerged and were responded to by both therapist and mother. Even though this approach explicitly avoids talking down to the parent, we believe it is also worth adding, whenever possible, positive statements about the parent's parenting, or comments that give credit to the parent for the child's positive attributes. These comments counteract the anxieties parents frequently have that therapists will negatively judge them. Such initial anxieties, present in family therapy of any sort, and with all families, become more acute in the case of child sexual abuse, in which the parent often blames herself to some degree.

The next few sessions followed the same format as the first. Through drawing and writing as well as talking, Sandra elaborated her feelings about both Mike and herself. She also explained her reasons for not telling her mother after the first incident: Her mother had told her that if anyone should touch her or try to touch her in her private parts, she should not let them, and she should tell her immediately. Because Sandra was too scared not to let Mike touch her, she was afraid to tell her mother. For months, she kept this secret, believing that she had done something bad. This shows how critical it is for children to be told clearly that they are in no way re-

sponsible for the abuse. When this occurs in an apology session with the offending person, the child experiences great relief.

Although Sandra did not tell after the first incident, when Mike
abused her again, her fear of him superseded her fear of her mother's anger,
and she told. Though Betty then spoke with Mike's "mother" (Linda) and
with Mike about the abuse, she had not talked with Sandra about the
meaning of the abuse for her. She had assumed (and hoped) that Sandra
would forget about it, and that as long as Mike stopped, things would be alright. Part of therapy alone with Betty centered on exploring the source of
these beliefs, which included the unfortunate assumption, based on her up-
bringing, that girls, as well as women, are often mistreated. During these
conversations, I learned that James treated her disrespectfully and had
maintained a long-term extramarital affair. Betty had asked him to talk
about their relationship, but he refused to, and would only say he was a
good husband because he was a good provider. When I asked Betty if she
wanted us to try to help her address her concerns with James, she was eager
to do so but doubtful that he would be willing. We agreed to wait until we
had completed our main goal of helping Sandra and Mike. However, we did
explore her assumptions about gender, and she began to question them.
She also began to consider that her daughter's future might be different
than that of the women she had known.

Working with Father and Son

I[3] began working with Mike in individual sessions, and with Mike and
James together. I focused first on strengthening the relationship between
father and son through helping them identify the blocks in their communication, which led them to talk more intimately than they ever had before.
Though James loved his son, and Mike knew it, the boy felt he could not
discuss the abuse or any other problems with him, because James would immediately become stern and endlessly lecture him. Indeed, the first session
with father and son, described later, showed this to be the case. Mike believed his father's behavior demonstrated a lack of real concern for him,
and James interpreted his son's tendency to "tune out" while he was talking
as a sign that Mike did not adequately respect him.

After first talking in an individual session about Mike's sense of being
alienated from his father, Mike and I discussed the upcoming conjoint ses-

---

[3]The therapist is Peter Fraenkel.

sion and how best to communicate his desire that his father listen to him more. In that session, when Mike described his feelings to his father, James quickly responded that his lecturing represented an attempt to protect Mike from the many dangers facing a young man. James, who had a long career as a foreman in a factory, went on to describe how he had watched helplessly as his brothers got involved with drugs. He was anxious and determined to prevent such an outcome for his son. Mike was visibly moved by his father's statements and said he had not known the depth of James's concerns for him. I built on this moment, noting that Mike spoke of wanting to express himself more fully to his father. I wondered aloud if James's lecturing, although well-intentioned, might block Mike from speaking and, in circular fashion, keep James from hearing what was going on with his son regarding matters that might need his fatherly guidance. James said this made sense and recalled that when he was a boy, his father lectured him often, and that, as a result, he found himself more likely to speak to his grandfather, who was more patient.

As sessions with father and son continued, it became clear that James held a number of negative attitudes toward women, and that Mike had absorbed some of these through observing his father. Although he respected his older sister Linda, James held little respect for younger women, including his wife Betty, with whom Mike was quite close. James also said he felt little responsibility toward her except financially. He did not see the need to respond to her requests for time together, talk, or monogamy. James noted that he had openly carried out relationships with other women, a fact known by the whole family. Although I attempted in a variety of ways to explore further his attitudes and their effects on Mike, James was quite firm in his views—at least as they pertained to himself. I then asked him whether he would view his son as less masculine if his son treated women differently. He said, no, that he did not think this would compromise Mike's masculinity.

Discussion

I began by working to strengthen the father–son bond and to open up their lines of communication for several reasons. First, given the concerns at the beginning of the therapy that James might potentially hurt or at least reject Mike, and his upset at having not been told about the abuse by the women of the family, it seemed wise to include him at the start of this phase of treatment. Second, I thought that discussing the abuse might be difficult for Mike, and because he already had his mother's support and permission to discuss it, I thought it would help to have his father's clear permission and support. Third, Marcia and I hypothesized that Mike's abusive behavior was probably facilitated by certain attitudes about men's entitlement to sex and an objectification of women, attitudes that in part he had possibly learned from his father. Therefore, I wished to engage the father to see if these attitudes came at least in part from him, and if so, whether he was open to exploring and modifying them. It turned out that James did model Mike's attitudes. Once these attitudes were brought forth, I could ask James if Mike had his permission to define his own way of being a man.

In continued individual sessions, I explored Mike's reactions to his father's view of women, then raised as a topic which ways he wanted to emulate James or, conversely, to be different from him. Mike, who was sexually active, reported with some embarrassment that one way he had come to emulate his father's interest in more than one woman was to make a game out of seeing how many phone numbers he could get from women he met on the subway. As we deconstructed the meaning of his behavior, Mike acknowledged that although this game made him feel "cool" and attractive, he really wanted a girlfriend, someone to get to know well as a friend, not just as a sexual partner. Through these conversations, Mike began to make distinctions that helped him clarify and define manhood in his own terms.

In addition, I suggested that Mike's current serious academic difficulties—he was in danger of having to repeat his junior year of high school, largely because he hadn't turned in homework—might be due in part to the amount of time and mental energy he expended on the game of getting women's phone numbers. He agreed, noting that he was generally preoccupied with "the chase," reducing his ability to organize his homework.

The discussions about how to be a responsible, caring man then led Mike to talk about the time when a man had been particularly irresponsible with him—when Mike was abused by his former neighbor. And once Mike was able to talk more freely and emotionally about his own abuse, he became better able to talk about his abuse of his sister. As we continued to talk about Mike and his sister, his focus shifted from himself and his upset about what he had done, and its consequences in terms of the family's reaction to him, to a more empathic focus on how Sandra must have felt. To expand upon this, I asked Mike to return to his memory of the abusive incidents, to slow down the action, and to imagine at each step what Sandra might have been feeling. I also asked the following more general questions: "Do you think it has affected her? How? How was her experience of being abused by you different than your experience of being abused by your neighbor?" As Mike considered and answered these questions, his emotional focus shifted from his experience to that of his sister.

In these sessions, Mike was also able to talk about the many women in his family that he loved and respected. In a subsequent family meeting with his "mother" (Linda) and James, he described these feelings, and they praised him. This support further assisted him to define the types of relationships he sought with women.

Discussion

This part of the work with Mike focused on connecting attitudes toward women and sex, and his own experience with abuse, with his abuse of Sandra. The conversation moved in an ever-enriching spiral from the micro-level of describing reconstructed memories of the moment-to-moment interaction between Mike and Sandra to empathy-building imaginings of how she might have been feeling, to discussion of his abuse-facilitating beliefs and experiences, and back again to the micro level. In this manner, Mike's tendency to objectify girls in pursuit of sex helped us understand how he could have depersonalized Sandra and overridden his own empathic cues to continue abusing her, and his growing empathy for how Sandra might have felt helped him to question his objectifying attitudes toward women in general.

When therapy ended, Mike had passed his courses and was headed toward his final year of high school. He had also stopped "hitting on" girls in the subway and elsewhere and was several weeks into developing a relationship with one teenage girl, with whom he wished first to develop a friendship, and only later, possibly, a sexual relationship. However, before therapy ended, we arranged a family session in which Sandra had the opportunity to hear an apology directly from Mike.

An Apology Session and a Safety Plan

In an individual meeting with Sandra, and then in a session with her and her mother, we discussed the idea of a family session in which Sandra could hear directly from Mike that he was sorry and took full responsibility for the abuse. Both Sandra and Betty liked the idea. After a session with Mike in which we discussed Sandra's wish for the apology, confirmed his willingness to participate, and went over Mike's apology to make sure he truly took complete responsibility, the family was convened for both the apology session and development of a long-term safety plan. Mike said to Sandra, "I'm sorry for what I did to you. It's not going to ever happen again, and it is my fault not yours. I am going to try to make everything 100% OK. I don't want you to be scared of me. I am not mad that you told, and if anything bad ever happens to you again, you should tell." Sandra just listened. We (Peter and Marcia) then suggested that the family develop a safety plan because, we explained, Sandra was still scared to be alone with Mike. There was then considerable talk among the adults about how to make it safe for Sandra to sleep over at Linda's home, where Mike lived. James thought she should just never sleep there, but Betty pointed out how much Sandra enjoyed being with Linda. After much back-and-forth discussion, the family decided that Sandra would sleep over only if Betty stayed there with her in the same bedroom. Marcia asked Sandra if she could tell her mother or father whether or not she felt safe. Marcia asked, "Could you say, 'I don't want to sleep there if Mike is going to be there?' Or would you think that someone would be mad with you, or that you might hurt someone's feelings?" Sandra responded that she could say it.

Discussion

Once Mike apologized to Sandra, we did not ask her to comment. We waited quietly to see if she chose to respond, but as we explained earlier, it is not the responsibility of the child who was abused to accept the apology or comment on it. We then moved toward working out a safety plan for her. Again, the emphasis was on the abused child's well-being. Though it can be tedious to work out the details of a safety plan, and tempting just to encourage the parents to develop it outside the session, it is essential that therapists allow time in session to consider fully all of the circumstances in which a problem could emerge that would put the child at risk for either fear or actual abuse.

Once the details of staying overnight were worked out, Peter asked how Mike's overnights at his father's home (where Betty and Sandra lived) would be worked out so that Sandra felt safe. The family not only worked on the details in terms of Sandra but also felt it was prudent to protect their young son, Teddy. Their conversation was quite lengthy and specific. At one point, Marcia asked Mike how he felt hearing this discussion about how to protect the children from the possibility of his abusing them. He responded, "It's necessary for them to feel safe. I know I'm not gonna do this again, but I can understand." Mike then went on to suggest refinements in the safety plan.

Discussion

Part of Mike's recovery centered on his increasing capacity to understand empathically the feelings and needs of others, and to demonstrate his ability to promote others' well-being even when this meant acknowledging shameful aspects of his own behavior. In his statement, he demonstrated confidence in his ability to control his impulses and a capacity to take on the perspective of others in the family. Because we did not prompt him to state these thoughts or feelings, we felt fairly confident, as did his family, that he meant them and could stand by them. In this session, Mike was empowered to be a protector.

Following the Apology

The following dialogue in a session 1 week after the apology captures the meaning that the apology session had for both daughter and mother:

MARCIA: So tell me how the last meeting was for each of you?

SANDRA: Good.

MARCIA: Good? In what way good?

SANDRA: Excellent.

MARCIA: Excellent? That good! How was it excellent? Could you explain, 'cause you are such a good explainer.

SANDRA: 'Cause he said he was sorry, and we all talked together.

MARCIA: (turning to Betty) Do you have any other ideas about why it would be important to Sandra that Mike say he was sorry and that it was his responsibility?

BETTY: I think she must feel relieved that it is no longer a secret. Even for myself, I feel that a burden has been lightened.

MARCIA: So you feel relieved.

BETTY: Yes, that it's out. She seems really happy to me. She even feels she is cute. Before, she was saying she was ugly, and now she says she is cute. She feels good about herself, and I'm feeling like the way you feel when you clean the house.

MARCIA: What a nice way to put it.

BETTY: Yes, I feel like we got the house cleaned up.

CASE 2: THE RELATIONAL BINDS
THAT SUSTAIN SELF-BLAME

The following account of a family in treatment illustrates how we use play to bring forth and loosen the relational binds that keep a child blaming herself for the abuse, even when she receives the full support of her nonoffending mother. These relational binds also keep her from experiencing and expressing her full range of feelings about the person who offended—the continued feelings of connection as well as anger and hurt at the abuse he perpetrated upon her. In addition, this account also demonstrates how relational questions, in this case introduced within a role-play format, bring forth organizing premises that prevent a child from healing.

Carmen, a warm, demonstrative 11-year-old Latina girl, lived with her mother, Dolce, in a small apartment in Spanish Harlem. Carmen was an only child. At the time Carmen began therapy, she was not experiencing serious overt psychological or behavioral symptoms but was having increasingly severe asthma attacks that frequently required hospitalization. We wondered if these attacks resulted in part from stress that she experienced following disclosure of the abuse.

Carmen's biological father, Joey, had abused Carmen regularly for 1 year, starting when Carmen was 9½ years old. Despite his abusive behavior, both mother and daughter described Joey as loving, kind, and fun. For example, because Dolce's social life was primarily centered on charitable work sponsored by her church, Joey took over all recreational activities with Carmen—going to the zoo, taking her to the movies, and so on.

Dolce, a rather timid woman, said that Joey's betrayal was beyond any description she could offer. Her stance, quiet but firm, was against having anything further to do with him. She had reported the abuse immediately upon discovering it, and at the time we met mother and daughter, Joey was serving a 6-year prison sentence.

In the first session with mother and daughter together, Carmen revealed how much she missed her father. She also repeatedly insisted that she was at fault for his being in jail. Though Dolce stated clearly that it was not her daughter's fault, Carmen did not budge from her position.

As the result of a Decision Dialogue, Carmen chose to bring the issue of her sense of fault for the abuse and for her father's jail sentence into the children's group that was ongoing at that time. Despite reassurances to the contrary from all the children, Carmen kept blaming herself. After a few such group meetings, Carmen was asked if she wanted to have an individual session. She accepted, and she and I[4] met alone.

In this meeting, I asked Carmen if she thought anyone else in the family blamed her. With no hesitation she said, yes, that her (paternal) grandmother blamed her. After hearing more about what the grandmother said to Carmen, I suggested that she and I do a role play in which she would play her grandmother and I would interview her. Carmen responded enthusiastically to this suggestion. The following dialogue shows how a therapist can use role play and humor to challenge a parent or grandparent's position, now internalized by the child, that she is to blame.

MARCIA: Hi, Ms. Lopez! How are you doing? (*Carmen smiles.*) I hear that you feel that it's your granddaughter's fault that Joey is in jail now for having sexually abused her. So I'm very curious. Would you tell me how it is her fault?

CARMEN: (*Has been playing with her bottom lip, but now sits up straight.*) Because . . . (*smiling*) . . . he wasn't responsible.

MARCIA: He wasn't responsible?

CARMEN: I think she would say that. I don't know. (*Leans back in her chair.*)

MARCIA: Oh, he wasn't responsible. Was he drinking?

CARMEN: I don't know (*shaking her head*).

MARCIA: Hmm. Did he have a brain tumor?

CARMEN: (*laughing, more relaxed*) No.

MARCIA: No. Was he on drugs?

CARMEN: No.

MARCIA: Hmm.

CARMEN: Not that I know of.

MARCIA: So why do you think he wasn't responsible?

CARMEN: Hmm (*tilts head to one side*).

MARCIA: He's a grown man.

---

[4]Marcia Sheinberg was the therapist.

CARMEN: Because . . . he's too young to understand anything.

MARCIA: (*leaning forward*) He's too young? How old is he?

CARMEN: Twenty-nine.

MARCIA: Did you say nine?

CARMEN: (*laughing*) Twenty-nine.

MARCIA: Oh, I thought you said 9. Because I couldn't understand—at 29 he's still too young to understand anything?

CARMEN: (*Nods.*) It was his first time being a father.

MARCIA: Oh. So you think he got mixed up with what was allowed?

CARMEN: (*nodding*) Yes.

MARCIA: So when you raised him (*Carmen looks up*), you didn't teach him right from wrong?

CARMEN: Yes I did (*emphatically*)!

MARCIA: So how come he didn't know it was wrong to do that? (*Carmen giggles and shrugs; I join her in laughter.*)

CARMEN: Because I never taught him about that.

MARCIA: You never taught him that it's not right to have sex with his daughter.

CARMEN: Right.

MARCIA: Well, do you think he knew that?

CARMEN: Umm (*shaking her head, no*).

MARCIA: I know you're his mother and you love him very much, and you want to protect him. Right? (*Carmen nods.*) But do you really believe what you're telling me?

CARMEN: (*Smiles, nods again, as if enjoying her stubborn role.*)

MARCIA: (*Laughs a little.*) That's very interesting. How do you think most first fathers know that they are not supposed to have sex with their young daughters—that sex is for grown-ups?

CARMEN: I don't know, but his daughter's responsible.

MARCIA: Now why is his daughter responsible?

CARMEN: Because . . . (*rubs eye, stretches*) . . . she was the one who put him in jail. She should have told me and not her mother.

MARCIA: Oh, she should have told you. And what would you have done?

CARMEN: I would have taken my son to Costa Rica.

MARCIA: And then what would he do there?

CARMEN: Stay in my house. Go to college.

MARCIA: So, you really don't think what your son did was very bad.

CARMEN: (*stretching arms over her head, again smiling*) Exactly.

MARCIA: Well, let me ask you a question. How will you protect your grand-daughter?

CARMEN: Well . . . (*plays with hair, stretches*) I don't know. But she is responsible.

MARCIA: She's responsible for what?

CARMEN: For sending him to jail.

MARCIA: OK. And who's responsible for what he did, that got her to tell the thing that got him to go to jail?

CARMEN: (*pausing for a second*) She is.

MARCIA: Why?

MARCIA: She—she started everything.

At this point, Carmen reveals that she believes she is responsible, because she thinks she initiated the sex between herself and her father. I inquire more specifically about the abuse and learn that, against her mother's admonishments, Carmen used to come out of the bathroom naked. Additionally, she explains that her father told her that if he should ever touch her, she should stop him.

Discussion

It seemed that her mother's admonishments about coming out of the shower naked, her father's instructions to stop him from abusing her, and her grandmother's anger because she disclosed, together convinced Carmen that she was responsible for the abuse. I decided to role-play with Carmen because, in direct conversation about the abuse, she seemed absolutely fixed on the one perspective provided by internalized blame. When I asked her who else might agree that she was to blame, her answer provided a direction that eventually helped me better understand her self-blame. Role play, like storytelling, puppet play, drawing, and other symbolic activities, is a medium that often suits children better than direct conversation (Gil, 1991). Given her level of cognitive development, Carmen had the capacity to enter a "debate" that eventually showed her the fallacy in her reasoning. Carmen engaged in the role-play debate enthusiastically. As I increased the absurdity of my questions in an attempt to challenge, with some humor, the tenacity of her views, she stuck to her position. When she ran out of answers to my question of why it was her fault, she revealed her more "shameful" belief—that she started, or at least encouraged, the sexual contact between her and her father.

Speaking directly to her, I asked Carmen how her belief might change. After a moment of reflection, Carmen answered that only her father's saying it wasn't her fault would allow her to feel differently. Asked if she had discussed these thoughts with her mother, Carmen said that she had not. In a Decision Dialogue, Carmen considered the benefit of discussing this with her mother. When I asked if she would also like to talk this over in the children's group, she declined. She preferred to speak with her mother but said she wanted me present.

The following excerpt is from our Decision Dialogue, which took place 1 week after the role-play session:

MARCIA: What I remember of our talk is that you hold yourself responsible because you feel that you started it, and because your grandmother blames you. And one of the things that I think you thought would help is if your dad wrote you a letter in which he completely took responsibility for it. Am I on the right track?

CARMEN: (*nods, and says softly*) Mm-hmm.

MARCIA: So, one thought I had is that we could talk with your mom about how important it is to you that your father let you know that he, and not you, is responsible. So what do you think?

CARMEN: Mm-hmm. It's nice.

MARCIA: Yeah? Why?

CARMEN: Well, maybe I can communicate with my father again.

MARCIA: You'd like that? (*Carmen looks away, and nods.*) You miss him?

CARMEN: Yes.

MARCIA: Have you talked with your mother about this?

CARMEN: No. I'd like to.

MARCIA: How would you like to do it?

CARMEN: Together with you.

Discussion

This dialogue well illustrates the relational context of beliefs about self. As has been frequently described in the research literature on self-concept, children's beliefs about themselves are highly influenced by the beliefs and attitudes held about them by the important adults in their lives (Mead, 1934; Harter, 1998, 1999). Carmen's belief that she was to blame could only change if she heard her father say she was blameless. In a sense, her father had to show he had fully internalized responsibility for the abuse before Carmen could release and appropriately "externalize" blame. However, this could not be a simple dyadic transaction; the relational context of this belief also included Dolce, who needed to support Carmen's wish to hear directly from her father—something that went against her resolve never to have anything to do with him again. Therefore, there was a risk that Carmen and I might present her wish to hear from her father and her mother might refuse. However, our sense was that Dolce would approve anything that helped her daughter fully recover. And even if Dolce did not want any contact between Carmen and Joey, her reluctance could result in an important discussion between mother and daughter that might promote a more open relationship between them.

In the family session that followed, Dolce was responsive to the idea that Carmen needed to hear firsthand that she was not to blame. Dolce concurred with Carmen's account that Joey's mother had blamed Carmen. Carmen then took this opportunity to tell her mother that Joey had laid responsibility on her to stop his sexual advances. Dolce came to understand the confusion Carmen was experiencing and appreciated how hearing directly from her father might help her. She even went beyond the idea of contact by letter and suggested that Carmen visit her father in prison.

The following dialogue is from the part of the session in which mother and daughter discuss Carmen's desire to hear directly from her father:

DOLCE: Well, I remember when a lawyer told us that when her father went to court, he said that he was the only one who was guilty.

CARMEN: But I wasn't there to hear it.

DOLCE: He was sorry about what he did.

CARMEN: But I wasn't there to see it.

DOLCE: Oh, you wanted to hear from him? (*Carmen nods yes.*) (*addressing Marcia*) Maybe she can go see him, and hear from him.

MARCIA: You think? In jail?

DOLCE: Yes—only one time. To hear that he's the only guilty person, that she doesn't have any of the responsibility, that she was a baby—nine years old.

CARMEN: (*objecting*) I was not a baby!

DOLCE: Yes. Nine years old, you were not an adult. You were too young to know.

Discussion

Dolce's decision was influenced by strong feelings of support and protection toward her daughter. These feelings changed her determination to keep her husband away from their daughter to a plan of contacting and including him in order to help Carmen view herself as blameless for the abuse.

Dolce decided to share her plan with others in the mother's group. After an engaging discussion that examined the possible benefits, risks, and alternatives of having Carmen see her father, Dolce decided it would be better for me to write to Joey and encourage him to write a letter in which he assumed full responsibility for the sexual abuse. Dolce and I agreed that the letter would not be given to Carmen unless her father assumed complete responsibility.

I wrote to Joey and told him about his daughter's therapy. I said that while he had caused her great harm, he now had an opportunity to help her begin to heal. He could do so by writing a letter to her in which he took complete responsibility for the abuse. I also explained that I would first read the letter and give it to Carmen only if I believed it would help her.

Discussion

If appropriately written, the letter would serve as a variation of an apology session (the usual format of which involves bringing the child, the person who offended, and the nonoffending family members together; see Chapter 7). In the apology session, the person who offended assumes complete responsibility for the abuse and demonstrates empathy for the child's experience. Given that we had no opportunity to assess the father's level of empathy and sense of responsibility beforehand, and would not be present at jail to supervise the meeting, engaging him to deliver an apology by letter rather than in person protected Carmen from further confusion about who was responsible. If her father did not assume full responsibility, we could correspond with him further and work on his ability to develop an authentic apology.

Joey wrote a letter in which he assured his daughter that he was completely responsible. He told her she was a wonderful girl and that what had happened was caused by him and him alone. He did not ask for forgiveness and wrote nothing that implicated her. His description of her, and his expression of love for her, was appropriate. He described himself as having a sickness and his jail sentence as fair. He was also clear that he wanted Carmen to have a good life.

I called Dolce to tell her that the letter had arrived and that I thought it was OK to show it to Carmen. She and I made an appointment as soon as possible, as we knew Carmen was eager to hear from her father.

When Carmen came to the appointment, I asked her how she wanted to read the letter—alone, with me, with her mother.

She said she first wanted me to read it to her, without her mother present. As I did, Carmen cried and said she was glad to hear from her dad. She also spoke about missing him.

After sharing these feelings, I asked her if she wanted to role-play again. She readily agreed, and I suggested that, this time, I would role-play her grandmother and she, her father. During the role play, Carmen, as her father, argued strenuously with his mother that his daughter was not to blame, that he was the one who did a terrible thing to his child.

We completed the role play and Carmen asked if we could read the letter to her mother. We invited Dolce in, read the letter, and then Carmen asked if we could do the role play for her mother to see. I agreed but suggested that, this time, Carmen play herself.

Discussion

Though Carmen had argued strongly in her own behalf playing her father, it was still in her father's voice, not her own. To argue in her own voice would indicate that she had fully internalized the belief that he, not she, was responsible for the sexual abuse.

In the following dialogue I am playing Grandma and Carmen is playing herself:

MARCIA: You did a very bad thing.

CARMEN: (*shaking her head*) No, I didn't do anything wrong.

MARCIA: You know you did. You told everybody that it was your fault.

CARMEN: There is nothing wrong or bad about me. It's all my dad's fault, not mine. I'm just an innocent little—girl. (*She smiles and looks toward her mother for emphasis.*)

Discussion

In this moment, Carmen drew upon her mother's description of her—"just an innocent baby"—and modified it to "innocent little girl."

Following this session, Carmen revealed for the first time the extent of the abuse she suffered. She quietly wept as she described the choices her father would give her, and told how she always chose the sexual act that would cause her the least pain.

Discussion

Acknowledging and responding to her attachment to her father allowed Carmen to move from being his loyal defender to openly feeling the anger she also held toward him. Whether coincidental or not, the frequency and severity of Carmen's asthma attacks dramatically decreased after this session.

CASE 3: STRENGTHENING THE MOTHER–DAUGHTER BOND

The following case history of a 9-year-old, Caribbean black child named Tanya and her mother, Cynthia, demonstrates key practices in the relational approach, including Talking about Talking, the Decision Dialogue, bringing forth the complex feelings of both child and mother, promoting personal agency, pointing the child toward a trustworthy family member, and helping the child not to blame herself. In addition, it is also an example of a child with at least a moderate level of trauma symptoms that are resolved mostly through relational work.

Tanya was molested by her 14-year-old cousin, Melvin, for over a year. The extended family was close, sharing child care, celebrating holidays together, and maintaining daily contact with one another. Children of various ages in the family played together regularly. Tanya and Melvin were born in a Caribbean country, and both families came to the United States around the same time, settled in the same area, and depended on one another for emotional as well as material support. Tanya's family was small, consisting of Tanya and her mother, Cynthia. Melvin's family was larger and included other siblings as well as grandparents.

Living far from other relatives, and estranged from Tanya's father, Cynthia was quite dependent on this large family. Therefore, the disclosure that Melvin had sexually abused Tanya was upsetting on a variety of levels. Melvin's family denied the abuse and was angry with Cynthia that it was reported. The abuse was discovered by Melvin's uncle and reported to child welfare by a pediatrician to whom Cynthia took Tanya after she learned about the abuse. The doctor explained that there was physical evidence of sexual penetration, and that she was obligated to report it.

Once it was reported, an investigation ensued in which a great deal of pressure was exerted on Cynthia to press charges against Melvin. The Corporation Counsel (prosecutor of juvenile offenders) threatened to encourage a neighbor—whose child Tanya had engaged in sexual behavior—to press charges against Tanya if Cynthia did not cooperate by pressing charges against Melvin. Ultimately, Cynthia decided not to press charges, because it would have required that Tanya testify in court against Melvin, and in her opinion, the experience would have been far too upsetting for Tanya. When we[5] began treatment with Tanya and Cynthia, the threat of Tanya being charged was still active and hung over the therapy like an ominous cloud until the Corporation Counsel agreed to withdraw the threat.

Though Cynthia (and later we also) invited Melvin and his family to participate in therapy, the family members refused, saying that they would seek help independently if they felt they needed it. They remained adamant that Melvin had not touched Tanya, and insisted that Tanya was known to lie. Cynthia repeatedly told them that she was not seeking punishment for Melvin, but that she wanted him to receive help. However, all her efforts were thwarted, and she and Tanya became estranged from the family. This rejection by the family was extremely hard on both mother and daughter.

We learned in the first session with Cynthia alone that Tanya was having recurrent nightmares about being killed by Melvin for revealing the abuse. Tanya had also described to her mother symptoms and showed signs of sexual hyperarousal, manifested in her engaging the younger neighbor in sexual activity. As we found out from Tanya in a later session, unbeknownst

---

[5]The therapist for this family was Marcia Sheinberg.

to her mother, Tanya was also preoccupied with the belief that her mother did not believe her account of how the sexual activity with Melvin had occurred; specifically, she worried that her mother blamed her.

We decided to work simultaneously on Tanya's specific trauma symptoms and the relational issues engendered by the abuse, thinking that they might be linked—particularly, Tanya's concerns about her mother not believing her and the loss of the extended family. Our hypothesis was that Tanya's symptoms would largely abate once she felt that her mother clearly supported, believed, and trusted her, and was ready and willing to soothe her. We sought to answer several relational questions: *Did* Cynthia blame Tanya for the loss of the family? If Tanya enjoyed aspects of the sexual activity, could she share this fact with her mother? And why didn't Tanya tell her mother? What blocked her—loyalty to Melvin, loyalty to her mother and a wish not to disrupt her relationship with the extended family, fear of her mother's reaction, or something else?

Discussion

Once again, it is our practice always to meet first with the nonoffending parent; otherwise, she or he gets too confused and inhibited about what to say and not to say in front of the child. Particularly sensitive to the impact of the loss of the extended family on Cynthia, I found that my empathizing freed her to expand on this loss and her sadness over failed efforts to create a bridge back to the family.

After speaking with Cynthia, I suggested inviting Tanya to the next session and engaged Cynthia in a Decision Dialogue about what we should and should not discuss with her. Cynthia was clear that anything she said to me could be shared with Tanya. When I asked if she thought it might be a good idea for me also to meet alone with Tanya, she readily agreed.

In the next session, mother and daughter reiterated the account of the events surrounding disclosure that Cynthia had described in our first session. Mother and daughter shared their sadness over the loss of contact with the extended family. When Cynthia asked if Tanya would like to talk alone with me, she said yes without hesitation.

Tanya was quite forthcoming, describing in a quiet, matter-of-fact way her bad dreams, her current fear of being killed by Melvin, and what she described as ticklish feelings in her vagina that make her want to be touched. After talking with her about these experiences, I described what we would do in therapy. I gave Tanya a notebook for writing or drawing her thoughts and feelings and explained that I would keep it just for her. We ended our first meeting together with Tanya and Cynthia agreeing that the next meeting would begin with my meeting alone with Tanya.

Discussion

The objective in the first family session was to develop rapport with Tanya and Cynthia together as a family. An additional goal was to create a context in which all thoughts and feelings were acceptable and safe to share. Whatever fears Tanya had about her mother not believing her, it seemed she experienced Cynthia's general support in the session, especially when she suggested Tanya might want an individual meeting with me.

When Tanya and I met the following week, I asked her if she would like to talk or draw her feelings about what had happened between herself and Melvin, and its aftermath. She chose to draw and write.

Discussion

Although we want to offer the child as much choice as possible in determining the content and process of any particular session, we are also clear with the child about the purpose of the therapy: to discuss her experience of the abuse. A nondirective therapy can create anxiety in a child who knows she is there because she was abused. Not addressing the abuse directly may also lead the child to believe that it isn't really safe and acceptable to talk about it. Like many other children, Tanya had not told any adult about the abuse before it was discovered. Therefore, from the outset, we wanted to clearly indicate that we were comfortable talking about it. However, if a child says she does not yet wish to address the abuse (through words, drawings, play, or other means), we honor her reluctance and suggest that it may be too soon. The therapist should not coerce a child in either direct or subtle ways.

Tanya decided to draw different pictures of herself. Underneath the drawings, she wrote the feelings captured by each facial expression: a "happy Tanya," a "sad Tanya," and a "frightened Tanya." Under the "sad Tanya," she described how she did not like it when Melvin put his penis inside her. As Tanya and I talked about this, it became clear she felt that there had been nothing she could do to stop Melvin, because he had convinced her that if she told someone, she would not be believed.

After helping Tanya elaborate on the experience, I asked if there were times when she felt differently than sad or frightened about the sexual activities with Melvin. Tanya then drew a happy girl and, when asked what made her feel happy, she laughed and said it was when he kissed her. I commented that it seemed there were times she didn't like it and times she did, and that she was clear about each. Using her language, I said, "You liked it when he kissed you and you didn't like it when he put his penis inside you."

Discussion

We never use more descriptive sexual language than that used by the child. By being matter-of-fact and using only the child's language, we communicate that we can absorb and witness her account of experiencing pleasure during the abuse without judging her. While some abused children have not experienced any pleasure during the sex, for those who do, it can create intense confusion and shame. Yet it is important not to elaborate the sexual description beyond what the child says, or else it can become arousing for the child, especially for one who is acting out sexually.

As the session progressed, Tanya described her fear during the abuse, which seemed to revolve more at that time around her concern that her mother would not believe her if she revealed it, than around the sexual activity itself. When I asked what led her to worry about this, Tanya explained that in the past she had lied when she thought she would get in trouble, and that her mother had warned her that people who lie are never believed, even when they tell the truth. She explained that she still thought her mother did not completely believe she'd told the truth about what had happened. Her fear was that her mother might think she instigated it. After exploring whether she herself believed this, Tanya said she didn't, but that Melvin had repeatedly said that if she told, no one would believe her. Tanya had linked Melvin's threat to keep her silent with her mother's earlier admonition. After Tanya's beliefs were brought forth and discussed, I suggested that her mother could let her know if she still wondered whether Tanya had lied, even a little, about what happened with Melvin.

Discussion

In this brief conversation, I encouraged Tanya in the next session to talk with her mother about whether she'd have believed her if Tanya had told her directly about the abuse, and to find out if her mother blamed her. I suggested this as a focus, because if Tanya continued to think that her mother doubted her account of the abuse experience, it might prevent her from turning to her mother in a future crisis.

Tanya decided that she did not wish to talk directly about this concern with her mother but preferred that I speak with Cynthia about it first. After this Decision Dialogue, I asked Tanya if she thought we had talked enough that day, or did she have other feelings she wanted to draw and discuss. Tanya said she didn't. I told her I thought she had shared a lot and I was glad that she did. I also said it was good that Tanya knew so clearly just how she felt, especially that she knew what she liked and what she didn't like. Tanya smiled hearing this and added that she liked it when Melvin treated her like a human being and didn't like it when he just did what he wanted to her. I responded that it sounded like Melvin was different at different times, to which Tanya said, "Yes, it's like he had different personalities."

Discussion

Asking Tanya if she had shared enough is an example of how we actively engage children to decide how much they wish to say, when they think they have talked enough, and to share thoughts about the therapy itself. It is important that this is not a pseudochoice; the therapist must respect the wishes of the child. Our effort is to create a collaborative relationship, even with young children. Therefore, we consistently seek opportunities for children to have a voice about the therapy process. Even small choices about the direction of the therapy or the direction of their lives help them develop an enhanced sense of personal agency.

This sense of agency is also strengthened by our comments on the child's acts of cognition, such how she distinguishes among various experiences or reflects on her preferences. For instance, when I commented about how Tanya distinguished between what she did and didn't like, the emphasis was not on the content (i.e., the sexual activity) but on the process of reflecting upon and knowing her own feelings. Once I highlighted this otherwise unnoticed example of her personal agency, Tanya elaborated these feelings in important ways.

As in working with adults, when children believe that the therapist accepts the myriad feelings and thoughts associated with abuse, they are more likely to elaborate them, discover additional ideas, and "hold" contradictory feelings. In order for the child to feel truly accepted, with all her mixed feelings and thoughts, the therapist cannot embrace this stance half-heartedly. The therapist must believe at a deep emotional level that all the child's thoughts and feelings do not have to be consistent, and that not everything can be synthesized and simplified. Like the family members with whom she or he works, the therapist must learn to live with the tension of irreducible contradictions.

When the family returned for their next meeting, I met first with Tanya and Cynthia together. Tanya quickly asked if she might read some additional feelings that she had written down after the previous week's meeting. She wanted to share them with her mother and me. Among the feelings and thoughts she described was a list of what she loved about Melvin. Also included was the language she had used in our discussion—for example, how she liked it when Melvin treated her like a human being.

Discussion

It seemed that once Tanya received the message that all her feelings were acceptable, she was free to allow herself both to risk sharing even more and to acknowledge to herself feelings that previously seemed unacceptable. For instance, her language changed from what she "liked" about Melvin to what she "loved." Furthermore, she shared the list with her mother. This demonstrates once again how important it is that the therapist not assume what a child may feel about the person who abused her.

Tanya read her list of feelings about Melvin. After listening intently to Tanya, Cynthia responded that she, too, liked Melvin. Cynthia then told of how, on her own initiative, she had called her relatives during the previous week and told them that she definitely believed Tanya. Tanya listened wide-eyed to her mother recount this conversation with the relatives.

After a few moments of silence, during which she seemed to be drinking in this important news, Tanya told her mother how happy she was that Cynthia called the other family members and took her side. This led mother and daughter to talk more about the cutoff from Melvin's family and how each was managing the loss "inside." After their conversation, I asked Tanya if she still wanted me to meet alone with her mother to talk about some of her worries. Tanya was clear that she expected this to happen. So Cynthia and I met to talk about why Tanya had not disclosed the abuse to her.

I began this meeting by saying that I was not clear why Tanya still wanted me to discuss this alone with Cynthia, especially since Cynthia had been so supportive—the phone call to Melvin's family being the most dramatic recent example of this. With a knowing look, Cynthia quickly responded, "I think she is afraid that I will lecture her. I used to lecture her when she didn't tell the truth, and tell her that no one would ever believe her again. I guess she might still worry about that." The conversation moved to Cynthia's beliefs about when it is and is not appropriate for children to speak directly to their mothers. This led Cynthia to talk about her relationship with her own mother. She described herself as very respectful of her mother and quite cautious about what she said and didn't say. Cynthia then reflected on the cultural differences between the country in which she was raised and the United States, where she was raising her daughter. She commented that she often thought children in this country spoke rudely to adults. Together, we explored the distinction between speaking openly and honestly versus rudely.

As our discussion about values and cultural differences deepened, Cynthia spoke candidly of how she particularly feared that her daughter would turn out like so many of her neighbors' children, and that instead of becoming successful, Tanya would start hanging out and doing poorly in school. Cynthia believed her daughter was bright and had great potential. We talked about how she tried to protect Tanya and how, at times, her best efforts backfired. I empathized with her aspirations for her daughter and shared that, as a parent, I had similar aspirations when raising my own daughter.

I then asked Cynthia if she was angry with Tanya for any aspect of the abuse. She was clear that she was not and that she held Melvin completely responsible. However, she was upset that Tanya did not tell her about it. This led us to discuss the reasons (in addition to fearing she would not be believed) that Tanya might not have told her about the abuse. The discussion provided an opportunity for me to talk about how we find that many children do not disclose to their mothers for a variety of reasons, and how this is understandably upsetting to a mother who wants to protect her daughter. I then asked Cynthia if she had talked about this with Tanya. She said she had tried, but Tanya did not respond; she just would get quiet. I asked if this was something that they might talk over. Cynthia thought this was a good idea, because she often felt frustrated when Tanya did not respond to her.

Discussion

In order to understand the relational blocks between a mother and her abused child, we invariably explore a mother's relationship with her own

mother and with other members of her family of origin, as well as the inter-
face between these relationships and the family's culture(s) of reference. In
this instance, I concentrated more on Cynthia's concern about the new
culture in which she was raising her daughter, as compared to the one in
which she was raised. I chose to express my empathic response to her and to
share similar, personal experiences as a mother for two reasons. First, because we were not able to hold a parent's group in the period during which
we saw this family, it seemed important to provide her with a sense that she
was not alone with her struggles—especially given how isolated she had become following the abuse's disclosure. Second, when we plan to address an
issue about parenting, a topic about which parents may feel defensive, we
find it reassures parents when we empathize with their challenges and the
positive intentions and goals behind their actions, even though we want to
suggest alternative ways that they might reach their goals.

In the next session with mother and daughter, Cynthia spoke to Tanya
about how she noticed that Tanya would get extremely quiet whenever she
asked why Tanya did not tell her about the abuse during the time it was occurring. Just as her mother had described, Tanya became quiet and lowered
her gaze to the floor. I asked Tanya if she could say what she was feeling.
She said being asked made her feel that her mother was not 100% on her
side. Cynthia said, "I can understand how you felt that I would not believe
you. I know I told you that once you lie, people don't ever believe you, but I
do believe you, and if anything ever happens again, I will believe you."
Tanya raised her head and met her mother's gaze. Mother and daughter just
looked at each other for what seemed like minutes—Cynthia, serious and
warm, and Tanya, intent, almost expressionless, but searching.

Eventually I broke the silence, noting that many children do not tell
for many reasons, and that maybe Tanya could use the chalkboard and list
some of the reasons she, like other kids, might not have told her mother.
Tanya went to the board and wrote, "Afraid my mother would be mad;
scared Melvin would hurt me; because everyone would believe Melvin and
not me." Cynthia said, "But didn't you know that because Melvin was
older, I would have been mad at him?" Now with full emotion in her face,
Tanya said, "Yes, but Melvin said he would say I made it up, and that I was
bothering him." With a gentle expression, Cynthia quietly said, "I see."
Tanya said emphatically, "I thought you would think I was lying like I used
to do!" Nodding with understanding, Cynthia said, "I guess you still worry
about that, but I do believe you." At this point, I interjected that even if
Tanya was "bothering" Melvin, Tanya's mother and I still held Melvin responsible because he was so much older than Tanya. Cynthia concurred,

and with this support from us, Tanya was able to describe in more detail how the abuse began and her confusion over whether it was her fault.

Discussion

A common worry among young girls who have been abused is that they may have instigated the abusive behavior by their "teasing," "flirting," "provocativeness," or simply by being affectionate or friendly. Once these worries are brought forth, parent and therapist can normalize these activities and clarify how the older person is still responsible. If the parent does blame the child, individual sessions can be used to explore and challenge the parent's premises that support holding the child responsible.

We often use a chalkboard when children are reluctant to speak. Sometimes children find it easier to write ideas and feelings than to speak about them. Using the chalkboard allowed Tanya to talk to her mother without doing so directly. It was a step closer than having me speak for her. After listing her reasons on the board, mother and daughter were able to talk more directly.

The conversation between Tanya and Cynthia continued for some time, with Cynthia clearly expressing her support and care for Tanya. I asked Tanya if she now believed that her mother was 100% on her side. Tanya said yes, and Cynthia reiterated how she felt completely on Tanya's side.

I then offered another explanation for why Cynthia wished Tanya had told her about the abuse sooner. I hoped my explanation might provide Tanya with another way of thinking about her mother's upset with her for not telling—one that would represent an alternative to Tanya's belief that her mother was not completely on her side. I suggested simply that her mother wanted to protect her. This explanation offered both mother and daughter a different way to describe Cynthia's reaction to Tanya's "not telling"—one that did not imply blaming Tanya and validated Cynthia's concern.

In a subsequent session, I asked Tanya how she was doing with her nightmares and whether she was still feeling the sensation in her vagina. She said she still had the nightmares, but less often, and that the tickling hardly happened anymore. I asked if she would like my help with either problem, and Tanya responded by suggesting that she could use a chart to keep track of when she had the nightmares and when she had the tickling, and for how long it lasted. I was so amazed by the clinical sophistication of this suggestion (as it is a common element of cognitive-behavioral treatment) that I asked Tanya if she "thought that up with her own good brain." Tanya chuckled and said she did. Then she drew a chart with the days of the week and column headings for each of her symptoms. When asked if she wanted to show her mother the chart, she said yes with pride and no hesitation.

Discussion

Although Tanya was clearly a bright child, she now felt empowered enough to generate and freely express creative solutions in therapy. Repeatedly, we find that as children develop and experience their personal agency, they amaze us with their resourcefulness.

When Tanya returned 2 weeks later for a session, she reported "no more nightmares" and in response to questions about her ticklish feelings, said, "I don't get them anymore."

Discussion

The content of this therapy focused less directly on Tanya's symptoms and more on the nature of her relationship with her mother, her different and contradictory feelings about Melvin, and clarification of her different physical and emotional feelings associated with the abuse. With this emphasis on resolving relational impediments to healing in a context in which Tanya experienced increased personal agency, her symptoms remitted with relatively little direct therapeutic attention.

Although it was important that the symptoms associated with the sexual abuse ended, we were concerned that when Tanya was older and experienced erotic feelings, she might regard them as bad or wrong. However, we also did not want to introduce this idea to Tanya at this juncture and possibly raise her anxiety or even renew the symptoms. We solved this particular therapy dilemma by talking it over with Cynthia. Whenever we have a dilemma about the direction of therapy, we discuss it with family members, and, inevitably, their input helps us resolve it. In this instance, Cynthia noted that she had already anticipated this issue. She had told Tanya that when she was much older and loved a young man, she would again feel these feelings, but that the feelings would make sense then, because she would freely have chosen to have them.

Given the absence of Tanya's symptoms and the now consistently open and supportive relationship with her mother, we all agreed to stop therapy for the time being. We set a plan that Tanya could let her mother know at any time if she wanted to come back, even just for a session or two. It was 8 months before I heard from Cynthia, who said that Tanya wanted an appointment because she had a videotape she had seen in school that she wanted me to see. When I saw her, she brought a tape that she had of an abused animal. She looked at me deeply and said, "Just like me."

Discussion

Again, because Tanya did not have the advantage of a children's group, she probably still felt that she was the only one who had experienced abuse. Her desire to share the tape and the important discussion we had about it has since led our treatment team to use psychoeducational materials, such as books, when we do not have a group. As with all elements of the relational approach, rather than providing such materials to all children at a particular predetermined point in the sequence of the treatment, whether and when such materials are introduced depends on the individual needs of the child.

Tanya and Cynthia continue to come to see me periodically. The calls are initiated by either mother or daughter.

Appendix A

Research Support for the Relational Approach

Although we have only recently begun a series of planned treatment studies (Fraenkel et al., 1998), much research indirectly supports the premises and practices of the relational approach. In addition, the relational approach provides a constructively critical lens through which to evaluate existing research. In this chapter, we first summarize the research on family risk factors for childhood sexual abuse; that is, we examine what research says is wrong with so-called "incest families." We then critically evaluate this research and argue that the notion of an "incest family" is problematic, potentially damaging to abused children and their families, and misdirects treatment. We then describe research on family and other variables that *mediate* the impact of abuse on children—factors that serve either to exacerbate or allay the effects of abuse. We end by showing how research supports our relational approach to child sexual abuse; how a relational approach can guide judicious clinical application of existing research findings; and how a relational approach can guide future family-based research into largely unexplored, clinically relevant areas.

RECONSIDERING RISK FACTORS FROM A RELATIONAL APPROACH

A growing body of research seeks to determine family risk factors believed to increase the likelihood of incestuous abuse. In this literature, families in which abuse

189

has occurred are sometimes referred to as "sexually abusive families" (Alexander, 1992; Howes, Cicchetti, Toth, & Rogosch, 2000), "incest families," or "incestuously abusing families" (Trepper & Niedner, 1996). As we discussed in Chapter 3, this language comes out of a traditional systems belief that problems such as incest play a function in the family, and that all family members contribute to circular patterns of interaction that maintain the problem (Alexander, 1985). This language and application of systems theory obscure the fact that incest is perpetrated primarily by men, who often believe they are entitled to obtain sex in this fashion and overtly or covertly intimidate not only the child victim but also the nonoffending female parent (Cammaert, 1988; Carter et al., 1986; James & MacKinnon, 1990). Even if authors note the need to consider the "individual pathology of the perpetrator" (Alexander, 1992, p. 185) in discussing the etiology of abuse, to speak of "incestuously abusing families" can unwittingly result in misattributing blame from the offending family member—whom we view as entirely responsible for the abuse—to other, blameless family members.

Furthermore, the body of work on family risk factors has not reliably established a particular family pattern, organization, or process associated with incest. Thus, although we agree with others who believe that research on family risk factors for incest and mediators of incest's impact will increasingly prove useful in treatment and prevention (cf. Howes et al., 2000), researchers and clinicians must remain extremely cautious in drawing conclusions from the current research, and must remain cognizant of the limitations of studies to date. Most important, we must remain clear about the distinction between family patterns that put children *at risk* of being abused, versus attributing the *cause* of the abuse to these patterns.

Risk Factors for Incest: The Current State of Research

Research on the risk factors, effects, and mediating variables of child sexual abuse is in its relative infancy, or at best, in its early childhood, well behind research on physical abuse and neglect (Crittenden, 1996). In order to be concise, our summary draws largely upon four excellent review articles and chapters (Berliner & Elliott, 1996; Crittenden, 1996; Kendall-Tackett et al., 1993; Knutson, 1995), and does not necessarily reference each finding.

Aside from the child's gender—females being at greater risk than males—and some indication that children with psychological vulnerabilities or disabilities suffer higher rates of abuse, especially those resulting in residential placement and direct physical management (Berliner & Elliott, 1996; Knutson, 1995), all four reviews point to aspects of the child's family and social environment as major sources of risk for sexual abuse.

In Finkelhor et al.'s (1990) retrospective survey of adults abused as children, the foremost risk factor to emerge was "growing up in an unhappy family" (p. 24). Similarly, conflict between parents or parental figures has been found associated with increased risk of abuse (Benedict & Zautra, 1993). In a number of studies, absence of or prolonged separation from a biological parent, or an emotionally distant relationship with a parent, have been found to put children at risk (Berliner & Elliott, 1996; Finkelhor et al., 1990; Knutson, 1995). For girls, living alone with the father or with two nonbiological parents were situations particularly associated with abuse, although all circumstances other than living with both biological parents were associated with higher risk (e.g., one biological parent and one stepparent) (Finkelhor et al., 1990). Boys were at inflated risk when living alone with their mothers or with two nonbiological parents.

However, these findings on the association between incest probability and family constellation are contradicted by the more recent NIS study that indicated children living in single-parent families, particularly when headed by mothers, were at no greater risk than children in other families (Sedlak & Broadhurst, 1996). Thus, no particular family constellation has consistently been shown to be more associated with incest than others.

Also, consistent findings have not emerged that pinpoint particular patterns of family interaction associated with greater risk of abuse (Crittenden, 1996). Hypotheses about "incest families" as more "enmeshed" or "disengaged," with unclear or rigid boundaries, poor communication and conflict resolution skills, poor affect regulation, unclear rules, or as characterized by a high degree of rigidity (cf. Alexander, 1985; Herman, 1981; Howes et al., 2000; Mrazek & Bentovim, 1981; Trepper & Barrett, 1989; see also a recent review by Trepper & Niedner, 1996) have received limited and equivocal support (Crittenden, 1996). Several authors have suggested that problems in the nature of the attachment between the nonoffending mother and child prior to abuse, and between the offending parent and child, may represent possible risk factors (Alexander, 1992; Crittenden, 1996). However, at present, these are merely interesting hypotheses without direct empirical support. Certainly, a growing literature identifies attachment difficulties *following* maltreatment (Cicchetti & Toth, 1995), but so far, there is little evidence that insecurely attached infants and children are more at risk of sexual abuse.

To date, the most striking and consistent findings—absence of the protective parent, prolonged separation between the child and the nonoffending parent, and emotional distance between child and parent—suggest that in these situations, the child is less protected by the nonoffending parent from exploitative family members and/or has less access or open communication with a protective parent. Thus, these conditions may be better viewed not as variables that represent qualities of an "incestuous family," but as problematic (in terms of abuse) only if associated with the presence of an abusive family member.

Limitations of a Focus on Risk Factors

The most obvious limitation of the current risk factor literature is the absence of empirical support for a particular set of risk factors. Of course, rigorous research in this field is relatively new and more work is needed. However, sometimes the tentativeness of findings is underemphasized in the rush to draw conclusions about the causes of incest.

In addition to a lack of consensus on risk factors, there are numerous methodological problems in studies to date that limit their validity.

1. *Few studies of children and families with appropriate matched controls.* Our comments here apply to the general state of research on abused children—on the psychological effects of abuse on the child, on mediators of the degree of these effects, as well as on risk factors. As illustrated by the contents of a landmark review article by Finkelhor and Browne (1986), prior to the 1980s, research on the effects of child sexual abuse largely centered on retrospective studies of adult victims recalling aspects of their childhood abuse, symptomatology, and family life. Few studies (4 out of 27 in that review) actually examined children and their families relatively close to the time of disclosure. A subsequent review (Kendall-Tackett et al., 1993) evaluated 45 studies of children and families, many of which were conducted during the 1980s and early 1990s. Most of these studies compared sexually abused children with nonclinical children or norms. However, as other reviewers have pointed out, still relatively rare in the empirical literature are well-conceived, matched comparison studies with adequate sample sizes that compare sexually abused children (and their families) with children who suffer from other clinical disorders or pathognomic experiences, and with children who have suffered other forms of maltreatment (Crittenden, 1996; Knutson, 1995). A recent exception is a study by Howes et al. (2000) that compared families in which there had been sexual abuse, families in which there had been physical abuse, families in which there had been neglect, and a nonmaltreating control sample. However, the generalizability of their findings is limited by the small sample (11 families in which there was sexual abuse) and because the sample was limited to poor families with very young children (ages 3–5). The interactional patterns of families in which children were abused during a developmental period in which parents are usually extremely involved and protective may differ widely from patterns of families in which the child was much older when the abuse occurred.

2. *Lack of a developmental model.* Cole and Putnam (1992) and Finkelhor (1995) note the atheoretical quality of much existing research on incest symptomatology and argue for application of a developmental perspective that would test hypotheses about the differences in impact of abuse at different developmental stages. The same can be said for the study of risk factors: Different family risk factors may be present or relevant at different stages of a child's development (Finkelhor, 1995; see also our discussion of Howes et al., 2000, above). Such a perspective would focus on assessing risks, effects, and mediators relevant to the particular cognitive, emotional, and relational tasks and abilities of children at different ages given that children's vulnerabilities and resources shift over time. The short- and long-term impact of incest on any particular child (and the activation of particular risk factors) may thus depend on where the child is developmentally at the onset of the abuse (Cole & Putnam, 1992; Finkelhor, 1995).

3. *Absence of prospective (follow-up) studies.* Also absent from the literature are

large-scale prospective studies that could better distinguish *risk factors* from the *effects* of abuse by following children and their families from the children's birth (or better yet, assessing families prior to the children's birth) through to children's adolescence and adulthood (Crittenden, 1996; Knutson, 1995). Such research would greatly improve on the current, questionable practice of inferring the risk factors that preceded and facilitated the abuse from study of the psychological and interpersonal characteristics of children and families *after* the abuse has already occurred. Research that infers preabuse risk factors from the characteristics of children and families reported and exhibited postabuse neglects the manner and degree to which the trauma of abuse can markedly reorganize the family's patterns of interaction (James & MacKinnon, 1990; Figley, 1989). In this sense, there is a curious incongruity in much of the abuse effects literature. On the one hand, the literature generally assumes that the psychopathology experienced by abused children is due to the abuse. On the other, disturbances of family functioning assessed at the same point in time (postabuse) are often assumed to predate the abuse and act as risk factors.

For instance, the retrospective finding that abused children have emotionally distant relationships with their nonoffending parents may not point to a preexisting risk factor but, rather, may reflect the anger and confusion experienced by both mother and child as a *result* of the abuse. As many of our clinical anecdotes have illustrated, distance between mother and daughter may follow from the abuse for a variety of reasons: as a result of the child withdrawing from the mother in an attempt to keep the abuse unknown to her because of threats from the offending family member, to protect the mother from the emotional pain of knowing, to protect the parents' relationship, or to avoid breaking up the family. Distance may follow disclosure of the abuse to family members because of the mother's resulting loyalty bind between child and offending partner, her not initially believing the child's report of abuse, the child's sense of betrayal because she was not protected by her, and so on. As Berliner and Elliott (1996) write, "Although it appears that families in which incest has occurred do exhibit greater dysfunction, it is possible that the pathology is at least as much a result of the incest as the cause" (p. 53).

In addition, retrospective risk factor research may underestimate the degree to which the abuse may negatively color how family members describe themselves at present or recall how they were prior to the abuse. Following disclosure, as family members themselves search for explanations for the abuse—in a sense, conducting their own assessment of the preexisting "risk factors"—they may magnify and latch onto negative qualities in themselves and each other that, prior to disclosure, might have been overlooked or incorporated into a more balanced picture that included positive qualities as well. Then, when participating in research postdisclosure, in which they complete questionnaires that ask them to describe family functioning, their responses may reflect this more negative view.

4. *Difficulty of disentangling antecedents from consequences in long-term cases.* An additional limitation of retrospective, postabuse studies of risk factors is that for

some percentage of children, the abuse may have occurred over a more extended period, long before it is disclosed. Even if the full extent of the abuse were known at the point of disclosure—often not the case, when the abuse has occurred over a number of years—it may be particularly difficult retrospectively to distinguish pre-existing risk factors from effects. In other words, with long-term abuse, how family members were prior to disclosure may be quite different from how they were before the abuse began, and to properly identify family risk factors, the relevant period is preabuse.

5. *Overlap between risk factors and effects.* There is often overlap between the problems that precede and follow the abuse. For instance, a child who has low self-esteem or little sense of personal agency prior to the abuse (a "psychological vulner-ability" that the offending family member may have exploited, knowing this child would be unlikely to report the abuse) may experience her self-esteem lowered even further by the abuse. As another example, a mother and daughter who are dis-tant prior to the abuse often become more so following the abuse (although some-times the abuse draws them together).

Practically speaking, whether or not there was preexisting emotional distance between the child and her mother, if there is such distance following the abuse, therapy needs to help mother and daughter to become closer. From the perspective of the relational approach, we are most interested in identifying the *current and fu-ture* risk factors particular to each family—both for continued abuse and for a poor adjustment following disclosure—and working in therapy to modify them. In fact, a number of studies addressing this issue have found that the degree of maternal sup-port of the child following disclosure appears to have a powerful influence on the child's recovery from abuse (Berliner & Elliott, 1996; Conte & Schuerman, 1987; Everson et al., 1989), as well as on whether or not the child is placed out of the home (Hunter, Coulter, Runyan, & Everson, 1990).

6. *Currently identified risk factors are neither necessary nor sufficient.* As research-ers have generally taken pains to indicate, the presence of any single risk factor alone does not determine whether or not abuse will occur. In other words, the current list of risk factors does not present a set of *sufficient* conditions for abuse to occur. For in-stance, even though the ratio of abuse by stepfathers versus biological fathers has been found to be five to one (Finkelhor, 1980), this does not mean that all stepfathers should be viewed as potential abusers, even when the family's situation includes a number of other risk factors as well. Likewise, the finding that girls who lived alone with their fathers, or boys who lived alone with their mothers, are at greater risk of abuse needs to be viewed as pointing to one possible, potentially facilitating environ-mental variable that in no way is established as a "cause" of abuse.

In addition, not all families in which there has been abuse have one or more of these risk factors. Thus, these factors are not *necessary* conditions for abuse; that is, abuse might happen even if these factors are missing. For instance, although we *have* at times found in our work with families a lack of closeness between the nonoffending parent (usually mother) and the child, this pattern is not inevitable (see also, Joyce, 1997). In one family we saw, the 8-year-old child had a close relationship with her mother, who had recently brought her older son from another country to live with the family. The 16-year-old boy had been repeatedly physically abused by his father, and, unbeknownst to his mother, was sexually abused on one occasion. The boy engaged his sister in "dry humping" several times before the sister told her mother. The sister, who had been raised by other relatives for several years in the home country and knew that the brother had been physically abused by the father, waited to tell her mother, because she didn't want to get her brother in trouble and have him possibly sent back to the father. Thus, in this case, an attempt to protect the brother, rather than lack of a close relationship with the mother, kept the child from reporting, and her relationship with the mother did not seem related to the onset of the brother's behavior.

7. *Differences in the meanings of risk factors for different families.* Two families in which there has been incest may share a similar set of risk factors, but the same factors may have different degrees of importance for each, depending on the particular significance or meaning of these factors, as well as the particular strengths and resources of each family. For instance, for a particular family in which the offending person was a stepfather, this may have more or less to do with the abuse depending on the degree of the stepfather's attachment to the child, at what age he entered the child's life, and many other factors. In other words, although it is useful to keep in mind the research and clinical data on generic risk factors as we interview a family, we believe that, in the end, we need to inquire about and treat the *unique constellation of each particular family's problems and experiences*—both those that have preceded and those that follow from the incest.

8. *The offending family member as the missing risk factor.* Another problem with the literature's conception and description of risk factors is that chapters summarizing them usually do not include a discussion of the characteristics of offending persons—even though it is widely recognized that the greatest risk factor for sexual abuse is the presence of a sexually abusive male who has access to a child. Rather, research on offending persons is usually presented in a separate chapter. In part, this may simply be due to the large body of research on offending persons, which might be difficult to summarize in a single chapter, along with work on abused children and nonoffending family members. However, researchers' and clinicians' tendency to separate discussion of factors that increase risk of *offending* from child or family *risk factors* may unintentionally contribute to and reflect a tendency to focus on preexisting problems with the child and nonoffending parent (usually, the mother), or the family as a whole, rather than putting the presence of a male prone to sexual abuse front and center as the major risk factor (Cammaert, 1988).

Summary: The Risks of Focusing on Family Risk Factors

As our review illustrates, *there is currently no clear empirical support for the notion that particular types of families pose more risk for sexual abuse than others.* As we noted in the Preface, Cole and Putnam (1992) write that "a specific preexisting familial dys-function has not been isolated" in association with incest (p. 175). Incest appears to occur in families of widely varying compositions and widely differing relational patterns. In addition, the absence of well-designed, prospective studies with appro-priate comparison groups makes it difficult, at best, to distinguish between family patterns that precede and increase risk for abuse and those that follow from abuse. Risk factors are neither necessary nor sufficient; any particular risk factor may carry a different meaning and weight for any particular family.

An additional problem is that a heavy focus on family risk factors may lead to ignoring sources of family *resilience*. Although, from a statistical point of view, risk factor research is in the broad sense "additive" in that it examines the additive or multiplicative negative impact of two or more risks applied to a family (Gerard & Buehler, 1999), philosophically, it is "subtractive" in that it examines family defi-cits rather than strengths. This deficit approach is not specific to the study of "in-cest families"—in examination of virtually all clinical phenomena, "few researchers have considered the family as a potential source of resilience—that is, as a re-source" (Walsh, 1998, p. 6). Where resilience has been studied, it has mostly been conceived as an attribute of the individual child rather than the family. Walsh ex-plains the history of this neglect of family resilience:

> Most studies of resilience have focused on children of a seriously disturbed or abu-sive parent; dismissing such a child's entire family as dysfunctional, researchers have looked for sources of individual resilience outside the family, in surrogate re-lationships—as with a teacher, coach, minister, or therapist—that counterbal-ance presumably destructive family influences. (p. 6)

Clearly, the notion of an "incest family" practically precludes interest in and identification of sources of resilience within the abused child's family that allow her a better recovery. In the following section, we discuss some of the aspects of the child's family and relationships that can worsen or lessen the impact of abuse.

WHAT MAKES THE EFFECTS OF ABUSE WORSE OR BETTER?

As we noted in the Preface, one of the most striking phenomena encountered in working with sexually abused children is that some children seem to cope fairly well, whereas others who experienced similar abuse cope much less well (Berliner & Elliott, 1996; Friedrich, 1990; Friedrich, Urquiza, & Beilke, 1986; Kendall-Tackett et al., 1993; Spaccarelli & Kim, 1995). Remember, also from the Preface, that a fair percentage of abused children even appear to be asymptomatic, with studies reporting rates between 21% and 49% of children with no symptoms

(Kendall-Tackett et al., 1993). (Interestingly, these findings replicate a 1985 review by Michael Rutter [cited in Walsh, 1998, p. 7] showing that "no combination of risk factors, regardless of severity, gave rise to significant disorder in more than half of the children exposed." We argued that children who do not show traditional signs of trauma or other intrapsychic and behavioral dysfunction likely do experience *relational trauma*— significant loss of trust in others and increased anger, hurt, and confusion about their family relationships, changes in beliefs about the safety of close relationships in general, and negative views of self *in relation to others* (as opposed to overall positive self-worth or self-concept)—that virtually no studies have assessed empirically.

However, it may also be that some variables mediate (increase or decrease) the likelihood that abuse will result in individual and relational symptoms. This section describes what is known about mediating variables. The research to date suggests that aspects of the quality of the child's relationships postdisclosure account for most of the variability in abuse impact. As we discuss, even mediating variables not deemed by researchers as "relational" per se make most sense when considered from a relational perspective.

Empirical Findings

As summarized by Kendall-Tackett et al. (1993), the strongest evidence to date suggests that more severe impact is associated with the following:

- Closer relationships between abused child and offending person. (See further evidence for this finding in a recent study by Ketring & Feinhauer, 1999).
- Greater frequency of abusive sexual contact.
- Longer duration of the period of abuse.
- Abuse that involves use of force.
- Penetration (oral, anal, vaginal).
- Lack of maternal support at time of disclosure.

Note that in this list of mediators of abuse impact, the first mediator is relational (the closer the abuser, the worse the abuse effects), the last one is relational (the closer the nonabusing parent, the less the abuse effects), and items in between make even more sense if we tack onto each the phrase "by a person whom the child trusted and loved." In other words, it is not just that a greater quantity of abuse causes greater symptoms (with "quantity" measured by frequency, duration, intensity, and intrusiveness); it's that these acts are particularly impactful because they are performed within a relationship that is expected to be the opposite of abusive.

Particularly noteworthy for our focus on family variables are the studies that link degree of maternal or other nonoffending parent support to degree of child distress following disclosure (Conte & Schuerman, 1987; Everson et al., 1989; Peters,

1988; Spaccarelli & Kim, 1995; Wyatt & Mickey, 1988). A study by Spaccarelli and Kim (1995) of variables hypothesized as influencing resilience to abuse found parental support to be the best predictor of freedom from clinical symptoms—better even than the total level of abuse-related stress, negative appraisals (defined as "perceptions of threat or harm related to sexual victimization" [p. 1174]), and active or aggressive styles of coping. Parental support was also the only variable significantly associated with another measure of resilience—the child's maintenance of social competence.

These findings echo those assembled in the broader developmental literature that indicate the central importance of family cohesion, warmth, and support in children's resilience in the face of stress (see review by Luthar & Zigler, 1991; Walsh, 1998). In addition, current work in the general area of child behavioral problems and psychopathology has increasingly addressed the impact of family interaction variables on symptom severity and type (Chamberlain & Rosicky, 1995; Estrada & Pinsof, 1995; Fauber & Long, 1991; Kaslow, 1996). As van der Kolk and colleagues write, "most children are amazingly resilient as long as they have caregivers who are emotionally and physically available" (van der Kolk et al., 1996, p. 432, references excluded).

Just as closeness of the mother–child relationship appears to affect recovery from abuse, closeness of the father–child relationship in the early years of the child's life appears to affect the likelihood of a father sexually abusing his child. Williams and Finkelhor (1995) found that fathers who had little involvement in the caregiving of their children were more likely to sexually abuse their daughters than were men who did more caretaking.

In addition to family mediating variables, there is an emerging literature on cognitive processing and its potential mediating effects on abuse impact. Berliner and Elliott (1996) reviewed this literature, and noted that, "higher levels of cognitive functioning are correlated with greater distress," and that "greater distress also is found in children who (a) have a global, stable, and internal attributional style, (b) blame themselves for the abuse, (c) view their experiences as threatening and use wishful thinking as a coping strategy, and (d) form various other negative cognitive appraisals regarding the abuse" (p. 61).

From a systems perspective, we would argue that even something as "individual" as the child's style of cognitive processing is learned, developed, and shaped within the family context, and that how he or she processes and copes with the abuse may be shaped by the manner in which the child's family constructs and processes events (see also Reiss, 1981; Walsh, 1998). Spaccarelli and Kim (1995) also highlight the relationship between the child's cognitive processing, active coping, and degree of parent support:

> Social support may protect victims by helping them to appraise what happened in a less negative way. In the absence of support, very few victims may be able to avoid making negative appraisals of themselves and of others. Active coping may

also interact with parent support, such that symptomatology is reduced when the victim tends to reach out in response to stress and the victim has at least one parenting relationship that is warm and supportive. (p. 1179)

Kendall-Tackett and colleagues (1993) note some limitations of the literature on mediational variables. First, studies that examine the degree of closeness of the relationship between child and offending family member typically only look at the offending member's kinship labels (father, stepfather, uncle) and do not assess the subjective degree of closeness or degree of regular contact, including the degree to which the offending family member was actively involved in caretaking. Second, fathers and stepfathers are often grouped together, which may obscure important differences in impact of abuse by a biological versus a stepparent. Third, a number of the intervening variables co-occur—for instance, intrafamilial abuse (involving a closer relationship between the abusing person and abused child) typically has a longer duration and involves more intrusive forms of abuse than does abuse by a person less close to the child. As a result, it is difficult to assess the independent impact of these variables.

Despite these limitations, research to date suggests that the critical positive mediating influence on the impact of abuse on the child centers on her relationship to a safe, caretaking other. In the next section, we discuss prominent theoretical models that illustrate what makes the effects of abuse more or less damaging. Again, although these theoretical models were not developed from a systems or (more broadly) family-centered focus, they buttress the case for such a perspective.

Relational Impact of Abuse: Theoretical Models

In two landmark theoretical papers on mediational variables associated with the type and degree of abuse impact, Finkelhor and Browne (1985, 1986) theorized about the central impact of betrayal on not only the child's intrapsychic and behavioral symptomatology but also her beliefs and expectations about relationships. According to this theory—largely based on studies of adult survivors, the dynamic of betrayal of the child by the offending person violates the child's belief that others will care for and protect her, and can lead to extreme dependence, clinging behavior, and/or mistrust; impaired ability to judge accurately others' trustworthiness; social isolation; vulnerability to subsequent abuse and exploitation; difficulties in adult intimate relationships, depression, and hostility.

From clinical data, Finkelhor and Browne also hypothesized that the nature of other dynamics between the offending person and the child would affect the intensity and pervasiveness of the impact of abuse on the child. These other dynamics include the degree to which the offending person encourages a sense of *powerlessness* by forcing and/or deceiving the child into sexual relations; a sense of *stigmatization* by blaming and denigrating the child for the abuse, and by pressuring her to keep the abuse a secret; and the degree to which he *traumatically sexualizes* the child by engaging her in premature and inappropriate sexual activity, rewarding her for this activity by exchanging it for favors, or for the attention and affection that would be due her based on their familial relationship; and by providing her with misinformation about sex.

More recent work has built upon and extended Finkelhor and Browne's original insights. For instance, Briere (1992) outlined the aspects of *psychological or emotional* abuse that occur as part and parcel of the sexual abuse, in the very nature of the abusive relationship of an offending person to a child, and sometimes in the response of the nonoffending caretaker. This abuse may include rejection, degradation, criticism, stigmatization, terrorization, isolation (through enforcing secrecy or keeping the child from social involvement outside the family), corruption (by cajoling or forcing the child to engage in sex), lack of parental responsiveness to the child's situation and pain, and unreliable or inconsistent parenting.

In his coping theory of variables that mediate the impact of sexual abuse, Friedrich (1990) also considers relational variables. While acknowledging the value of Finkelhor's model, Friedrich noted that it is largely focused on the child's "initial cognitive appraisal" of the abuse and leaves out many other variables that potentially mediate the impact of the abuse. In particular, his model considers the continuing impact of the quality of the child's interactions with family members and with the larger system (school, social services, court); the coping abilities of all family members; the child's intrapsychic development; and the role of triggering events, such as the movement into adolescence, a loss, and other life transitions and experiences. Likewise, Spaccarelli's (1994) transactional model of the impact of sexual abuse regards the quality of the child's familial and other relationships as critical to whether or not the child becomes distressed or develops overt behavioral symptoms.

DIRECTIONS FOR FUTURE RESEARCH FROM A RELATIONAL PERSPECTIVE

Research to date has largely conceptualized "impact" in terms of symptoms suffered by the child (depression, fear, anxiety, somatic complaints, lowered self-esteem) and problem behaviors (aggression, school difficulties, sexualized behavior). Although researchers recognize that these symptoms and behaviors may affect the child's interactions with family, peers, and others, study of these abuse sequelae has proceeded largely from a "problem-is-in-the-individual," nonsystemic, traditional diagnostic paradigm. As a result, little research has directly explored the possible circular, recursive relationships between the child's symptomatology, resilience, and the specific reactions of other family members to the child and among themselves.

From a systems perspective, a problem that is viewed as "located" primarily "in" an individual will affect and be affected by the other levels of the system. For example, a child's traumatic memories or nightmares (individual level) may affect the feelings of her nonoffending parent and siblings (individual levels) and the relationships among these family members (e.g., the child's symptoms may draw the mother closer in her attempts to care for the child, or may lead the mother to distance herself from the child out of fear, annoyance, or a sense of ineffectiveness). In turn, the quality of the mother–daughter interaction around the child's symptoms may affect the intensity of the symptoms. The child's symptoms may also affect her relationship to larger systems (e.g., when she is tired and doing poorly in school because of flashbacks and loss of sleep), and this relationship may either increase the negative effects of the symptoms (e.g., when teachers do not know why the child is doing poorly and blame it on low motivation) or decrease them (e.g., when a teacher takes special interest in helping the child do her best).

Future research on the relational impact of abuse needs to move beyond simple dyadic conceptions to examine the complexities of the relationships among the child, offending and nonoffending parents, other family members, and other persons (neighbors, teachers) involved with the family. Furthermore, the research needs to examine the *reciprocal connection* between the abuse and the child's relationships. To date, most of the conceptualization and research has adopted a more linear view—for instance, examining the impact of the quality of the child's relationships on the degree to which the abuse affects her, without at the same time including a focus on the impact of the abuse on those relationships, which in turn may affect the quality and degree of support given to the child.

Although research on mediating variables does address the impact on child recovery of such variables as parental support (Berliner & Elliott, 1996; Conte & Schuerman, 1987; Everson et al., 1989; Spaccarelli & Kim, 1995), virtually no research has explored this empirical relationship in detail. For instance, research is needed to identify which expressions and types of parental support (believing the child's account vs. talking with the child about the abuse, offering verbal reassurance and physical comforting vs. offering a structuring environment that encourages the child to return to normal daily activities) are most effective in general, or whether particular types of support are more helpful for particular types of child problems or at particular times. Spaccarelli and Kim (1995) note that "in some cases, a high level of parental concern about the abuse can lead to parental behaviors that are intended to be supportive, but fail to have a positive effect on the relationship or the victims' symptomatology" (p. 1180). They note the need "to empirically document the kinds of interactions that are critical to effective support after disclosure of sexual abuse" (p. 1180). Another question for future research is whether parents have an easier time supporting children who present with certain symptoms (e.g., anxiety or depression) versus others (sexualized or aggressive behavior), as well as the complex interplay between the child's temperament and the parent's emotional readiness to provide support (Luthar & Zigler, 1991). A further question centers on how the degree of distress experienced by the nonoffending parent about the abuse and its disclosure—distress that may be considerable (Deblinger & Heflin, 1996)—affects her ability to support the child.

In addition, little research has tackled the critical clinical question of which systemic, relational variables facilitate or impede parental support of the child: In other words, how the nature of the nonoffending parent's relationships with other family members (including the offending person, her own parents and grandparents), as well as the more complex triangles and interstices among the nonoffending parent, the child, and other family members, may affect her ability to offer the child support. To date, the research suggests that "the closer the relationship of the offender to the mother, the more likely that support will be compromised" (Berliner & Elliott, 1996, p. 61). However, as we noted earlier, much of the research to date defines "closeness" only in terms of kinship relation, not in terms of the more subtle aspects of emotional closeness. Much more needs to be learned about what it is about the nature of the *emotional closeness* between nonoffending parent and offending family member that impedes support for the child, as well as which factors distinguish those nonoffending parents who support their children—despite being "close" to the offending family member—from those who do not. In the preceding chapters, we have described some of our hypotheses about the role of complex attachments between the nonoffending parent and the offending partner or child that we believe impede the nonoffending parent's ability to protect her child.

From a systemic vantage point, in order to understand both the variability in children's responses to abuse and their recovery, we believe it is critical to understand the impact of the abuse and its disclosure on the family as a whole, on particular relationships within the family, as well as on the relationships between the family and its community (including neighbors, friends, the child's school, the family's religious community, and the professionals involved postdisclosure). The child's and family's experiences are embedded in, affect, and are affected by their social context. The need to look not only at relationships within the family but also at family members' access to a broader social network gains support from the broader literature on resilience, which views degree of use of support systems as a major category of variables associated with successful coping with stress (Garmezy, 1985; Luthar & Zigler, 1991; Walsh, 1998).

Put another way, much more work is needed to understand the variables that *mediate the mediating variables*—especially those that affect the degree to which a parent offers support for the child following disclosure. In addition, research needs to examine the efficacy of interventions that focus on strengthening the nonoffending parent–child bond (Spaccarelli & Kim, 1995).

The relative paucity of studies in the abuse effects literature of not only abuse-related changes in the *child's* experience of family members, but also of the impact of the abuse on all of the family members' relationships is particularly striking given the general agreement in the field that a major source of the negative sequelae of intrafamilial sexual abuse is the *betrayal and violation of trust in a familial relationship*. For instance, Cole and Putnam (1992) write, "Although child sexual abuse is a form of trauma, incest by a father is rarely a discrete traumatic event. In its most typical form, the abuse is a disturbance in an existing primary relationship that has as its focal points episodes of unwanted sexual contact" (p. 174). And Berliner and Elliott (1996) write, "Fundamentally, the harm can be attributed to the fact that sexual abuse is always nonconsensual . . . and invariably alters the nature of the relationship within which it occurs" (p. 55). Thinking more broadly than about sexual abuse alone, Cicchetti (1989) has described maltreatment as "relational psychopathology," and a recently published first comprehensive text on relational diagnosis includes a chapter on intrafamilial child sexual abuse (Trepper & Niedner, 1996). In addition, research on the long-term (adult) impact of abuse documents the negative effects of abuse on many survivors' capacities for close relationships, and on their often negative views of themselves and their families of origin (Berliner & Elliott, 1996; Cole & Putnam, 1992).

In the absence of many empirical findings on children's and families' experiences closer to the time of the abuse, we must at this juncture rely on theory, clinical impressions, and studies of adult survivors to outline the possible "immediate" *relational* impact of incest on abused *children* and other family members. In this book, we have detailed our approach to clinical intervention based on these relational effects of abuse, an approach that highlights the relational resources and resilience of families.

Appendix B

Information on Child Sexual Abuse

The following organizations provide a variety of types of information and other resources related to child abuse and neglect, including sexual abuse. This is a representative, but not exhaustive, list.

American Professional Society on the Abuse of Children (APSAC)
407 South Dearborn, Suite 1300
Chicago, IL 60605
(312) 554-0166
E-mail: *apsacmems@aol.com*
Web Site: *www.apsac.org*

The Brooklyn Child Advocacy Center (CAC)[1]
30 Main Street
Brooklyn, NY 11201
(718) 260-6080
Fax: (718) 260-6083
E-mail: *jwinston@victimservices.org*

---

[1]There are child advocacy centers in many states. This is an excellent example of what such centers offer.

International Society for Traumatic Stress Studies (ISTSS)
60 Revere Drive, Suite 500
Northbrook, IL 60062
(847) 480-9028
E-mail: *istss@istss.org*
Web Site: *www.istss.org*

National Children's Advocacy Center (NCAC)
200 Westside Square, Suite 700
Huntsville, AL 35801
(256) 533-0531
Fax: (256) 534-6883
E-mail: *webmaster@mcac-hsv.org*
Web Site: *www.ncac-hsv.org*

National Clearinghouse on Child Abuse and Neglect Information (NCCAN)
National Center on Child Abuse and Neglect
330 C Street, SW
Washington, DC 20477
(800) 394-3366 or (703) 385-7565
Fax: (703) 385-3206
E-mail: *nccanch@calib.com*
Web Site: *www.calib.com/nccanch*

National Data Archive on Child Abuse and Neglect (NDACAN)
Family Life Development Center—MVR Hall
Cornell University
Ithaca, NY 14853
(607) 255-7799
E-mail: *ndacan@cornell.edu*
Web Site: *www.ndacan.cornell.edu*

National Resources on Child Sexual Abuse

	APSAC	CAC	ISTSS	NCAC	NCCAN	NDACAN
Community education and training	×	×		×		×
Professional education and training		×		×		
Conferences	×	×	×			×
Discussion forums			×			
Internet discussion groups						×
Assessment and treatment of abused children		×				
Child forensics interviewing clinic	×	×				
Volunteer programs		×				
Epidemiological information		×			×	×
National incidence reports					×	
Journal	×		×			
Newsletter		×	×			×
Handbook and/or manual	×				×	×
Fact sheets		×			×	×
Information packets		×	×			
Prevention resources	×				×	
Other publications	×				×	
Resource listings		×	×	×	×	×
Internship programs		×				

References

Alexander, P. C. (1985). A systems theory conceptualization of incest. *Family Process, 24,* 79–88.

Alexander, P. C. (1992). Application of attachment theory to the study of sexual abuse. *Journal of Consulting and Clinical Psychology, 60,* 185–195.

Belsky, J., Rovine, M., & Fish, M. (1989). The developing family system. In M. R. Gunnar & E. Thelen (Eds.), *Minnesota Symposia on Child Psychology: Vol. 22. Systems and development* (pp. 119–166). Hillsdale, NJ: Erlbaum.

Bengis, S. (1997). Comprehensive service delivery with a continuum of care. In G. Ryan & S. Lane (Eds.), *Juvenile sexual offending* (2nd ed., pp. 211–218). San Francisco: Jossey-Bass.

Benjamin, J. (1988). *The bonds of love.* New York: Pantheon Books.

Bentovim, A. (1998). A full circle: Psycho-dynamic understanding and systems theory. *Journal of Family Therapy, 20,* 113–122.

Bentovim, A., Elton, A., Hildebrand, J., Tranter, M., & Vizard, E. (Eds.). (1988). *Child sexual abuse within the family.* London: Wright.

Bergman, S. J., & Surrey, J. (1994). *Couples therapy: A relational approach.* Wellesley, MA: Stone Center.

Berliner, L. L., & Elliot, D. M. (1996). Sexual abuse of children. In J. Briere, L. Berliner, J. A. Bulkley, C. Jenny, & T. Reid (Eds.), *The APSAC handbook on child maltreatment* (pp. 51–71). Thousand Oaks, CA: Sage.

Berliner, L., & Rawlings, L. (1991). *A treatment manual for children's sexual behavior problems.* Unpublished manuscript, Harborview Sexual Assault Center, Seattle, WA.

207

Benedict, L. L., & Zautra, A. A. (1993). Family environment characteristics as risk factors for child sexual abuse. *Journal of Consulting and Clinical Psychology, 22,* 365–374.

Boszormenyi-Nagy, I., & Spark, G. L. (1973). *Invisible loyalties: Reciprocity in intergenerational family therapy.* New York: Harper & Row.

Brickman, J. (1984). Feminist, nonsexist, and traditional models of therapy: Implications for working with incest. *Women and Therapy, 3,* 49–67.

Briere, J. (1992). *Child abuse trauma: Theory and treatment of lasting effects.* Newbury Park, CA: Sage.

Butler, J. (1990). *Gender trouble.* New York: Routledge.

Byng-Hall, J. (1995). Creating a secure family base: Some implications of attachment theory for family therapy. *Family Process, 34,* 45–58.

Cammaert, L. P. (1988). Nonoffending mothers: A new conceptualization. In L. E. Walker (Ed.), *Handbook on sexual abuse of children: Assessment and treatment issues* (pp. 309–325). New York: Springer.

Carter, B., Papp, P., Silverstein, O., & Walters, M. (1986). The Procrustean Bed. *Family Process, 25,* 301–304.

Chamberlain, P., & Rosicky, J. G. (1995). The effectiveness of family therapy in the treatment of adolescents with conduct disorders and delinquency. *Journal of Marital and Family Therapy, 21,* 441–460.

Cicchetti, D. (1989). How research on maltreatment has informed the study of child development: Perspectives from developmental psychopathology. In D. Cicchetti & V. Carlson (Eds.), *Child maltreatment: Theory and research on the causes and consequences of child abuse and neglect* (pp. 377–431). New York: Cambridge University Press.

Cicchetti, D., & Toth, S. L. (1995). A developmental psychopathology perspective on child abuse and neglect. *Journal of the American Academy of Child and Adolescent Psychiatry, 34,* 541–565.

Chodorow, N. (1978). *The reproduction of mothering: Psychoanalysis and the sociology of gender.* Berkeley: University of California Press.

Cohen, J. A., & Mannarino, A. P. (1993). A treatment model for sexually abused preschoolers. *Journal of Interpersonal Violence, 8,* 115–131.

Colapinto, J. A. (1995). Dilution of family process in social services: Implications for treatment of neglectful families. *Family Process, 34,* 59–74.

Cole, P. M., & Putnam, F. W. (1992). Effect of incest on self and social functioning: A developmental psychopathology perspective. *Journal of Consulting and Clinical Psychology, 60,* 174–184.

Conte, J. R. (1984). Progress in treating the sexual abuse of children. *Social Work, 29,* 258–263.

Conte, J. R., & Schuerman, J. R. (1987). Factors associated with an increased impact of child sexual abuse. *Child Abuse and Neglect, 11,* 201–211.

Crittenden, P. M. (1996). Research on maltreating families: Implications for intervention. In J. Briere, L. Berliner, J. A. Bulkley, C. Jenny, & T. Reid (Eds.), *The APSAC handbook on child maltreatment* (pp. 158–174). Thousand Oaks, CA: Sage.

Davies, J. M., & Frawley, M. G. (1994). *Treating the adult survivor of childhood sexual abuse*. New York: Basic.

de Beauvior, S. (1974). *The second sex*. New York: Vintage Books.

Deblinger, E., & Heflin, A. (1996). *Treating sexually abused children and their nonoffending parents: A cognitive-behavioral approach*. Thousand Oaks, CA: Sage.

Donley, M. G. (1993). Attachment and the emotional unit. *Family Process, 32*, 3–20.

Efran, J. S., & Clarfield, L. E. (1992). Constructionst therapy: Sense and nonsense. In S. McNamee & K. J. Gergen (Eds.), *Therapy as social construction* (pp. 200–217). London: Sage.

Elliott, D. M., & Briere, J. (1994). Forensic sexual abuse evaluations: Disclosures and symptomatology. *Behavioral Sciences and the Law, 12*, 261–277.

Elms, R. (1990). Hostility, apathy, silence, and denial: Inviting abusive adolescents to argue for change. In M. Durrant & C. White (Eds.), *Ideas for therapy with sexual abuse* (pp. 111–131). Adelaide, Australia: Dulwich Centre Publications.

Estrada, A. U., & Pinsof, W. M. (1995). The effectiveness of family therapies for selected behavioral disorders of childhood. *Journal of Marital and Family Therapy, 21*, 403–440.

Everson, M. D., Hunter, W. M., Runyan, D. K., Edelsohn, G. A., & Coulter, M. L. (1989). Maternal support following disclosure of incest. *American Journal of Orthopsychiatry, 59*, 198–207.

Falicov, C. J. (1995). Training to think culturally: A multidimensional comparative framework. *Family Process, 34*, 373–388.

Fauber, R. L., & Long, N. (1991). Children in context: The role of the family in child psychotherapy. *Journal of Consulting and Clinical Psychology, 59*, 813–820.

Figley, C. R. (1989). *Helping traumatized families*. San Francisco: Jossey-Bass.

Finkelhor, D. (1979). *Sexually victimized children*. New York: Free Press.

Finkelhor, D. (1980). Risk factors in the sexual victimization of children. *Child Abuse and Neglect, 4*, 265–273.

Finkelhor, D. (1994). The international epidemiology of child sexual abuse. *Child Abuse and Neglect, 18*, 409–417.

Finkelhor, D. (1995). The victimization of children: A developmental perspective. *American Journal of Orthopsychiatry, 65*, 177–193.

Finkelhor, D., & Browne, A. (1985). The traumatic impact of child sexual abuse: A conceptualization. *American Journal of Orthopsychiatry, 55*, 530–541.

Finkelhor, D., & Browne, A. (1986). Initial and long-term effects: A conceptual framework. In D. Finkelhor & Associates, *A sourcebook on child sexual abuse* (pp. 180–198). Newbury Park, CA: Sage.

Finkelhor, D., & Hotaling, G. T. (1984). Sexual abuse in the National Incidence Study of Child Abuse and Neglect: An appraisal. *Child Abuse and Neglect, 8*, 23–33.

Finkelhor, D., Hotaling, G., Lewis, I. A., & Smith, C. (1990). Sexual abuse in a national survey of adult men and women: Prevalence, characteristics, and risk factors. *Child Abuse and Neglect, 14*, 19–28.

Fraenkel, P. (1994). *The Therapy Experiences Scale.* Unpublished scale, Ackerman Institute for the Family, New York, NY.

Fraenkel, P. (1995). The nomothetic–idiographic debate in family therapy. *Family Process, 34*, 113–121.

Fraenkel, P. (1997). Systems approaches to couple therapy. In W. K. Halford & H. Markman (Eds.), *Clinical handbook of marriage and couple interventions* (pp. 379–413). London: Wiley.

Fraenkel, P., & Pinsof, W. (in press). Teaching family therapy-centered integration: Assimilation and beyond. *Journal of Psychotherapy Integration.*

Fraenkel, P., Schoen, S., Perko, K., Mendelson, T., Kushner, S., & Islam, S. (1998). The family speaks: Family members' descriptions of therapy for sexual abuse. *Journal of Systemic Therapies, 17*, 39–60.

Fraenkel, P., Sheinberg, M., & True, F. (1996). *Making families safe for children: Handbook for a family-centered approach to intrafamilial child sexual abuse.* New York: Ackerman Institute for the Family.

Freedman, J., & Combs, G. (1996). *Narrative therapy: The social construction of preferred realities.* New York: Norton.

Friedrich, W. N. (1990). *Psychotherapy of sexually abused children and their families.* New York: Norton.

Friedrich, W. N. (1995). *Psychotherapy with sexually abused boys: An integrated approach.* Thousand Oaks, CA: Sage.

Friedrich, W. N., Urquiza, A. J., & Beilke, R. L. (1986). Behavior problems in sexually abused young children. *Journal of Pediatric Psychology, 11*, 47–57.

Garmezy, N. (1985). Stress-resistant children: The search for protective factors. In J. E. Stevenson (Ed.), *Recent research in developmental psychopathology* (pp. 113–233). Oxford, England: Pergamon Press.

Gelinas, D. J. (1988). Family therapy: Characteristic family constellation and basic therapeutic stance. In S. M. Sgroi (Ed.), *Vulnerable populations: Evaluation and treatment of sexually abused children and adult survivors* (Vol. 1, pp. 25–49). New York: Lexington Books.

Gerard, J. M., & Buehler, C. (1999). Multiple risk factors in the family environment and youth problem behaviors. *Journal of Marriage and the Family, 61*, 343–361.

Gergen, K. J. (1985). The social constructionist movement in modern psychology. *American Psychologist, 40*, 266–275.

Gergen, K. J. (1991). *The saturated self: Dilemmas of identity in contemporary life.* New York: Basic Books.

Gil, E. (1991). *The healing power of play: Working with abused children.* New York: Guilford Press.

Gil, E. (1996). *Treating abused adolescents.* New York: Guilford Press.

Gil, E., & Johnson, T. C. (1993). *Sexualized children: Assessment and treatment of sexualized children and children who molest.* Rockville, MD: Launch Press.

Gilligan, C., Ward, J. V., & Taylor, M. J., with Bardige, B. (1988). *Mapping the moral domain.* Cambridge, MA: Harvard University Press.

Goldner, V. (1993). Current trends in feminist thought and therapy. *Journal of Feminist Family Therapy, 4,* 73–83.

Goldner, V. (1998). The treatment of violence and victimization in intimate relationships. *Family Process, 37,* 263–286.

Goldner, V. (1999). Morality and multiplicity: Perspectives on the treatment of violence in intimate life. *Journal of Marital and Family Therapy, 25,* 325–336.

Goldner, V., Penn, P., Sheinberg, M., & Walker, G. (1990). Love and violence: Gender paradoxes in volatile attachments. *Family Process, 29,* 343–364.

Greenberg, J., & Mitchell, S. (1983). *Object relations in psychoanalytic theory.* Cambridge, MA: Harvard University Press.

Haley, J. (1963). *Strategies of psychotherapy.* New York: Grune & Stratton.

Hare-Mustin, R. T., & Marecek, J. (1994). Feminism and postmodernism: Dilemmas and points of resistance. *Dulwich Centre Newsletter, 4,* 13–19.

Harter, S. (1987). The determinants and mediational role of global self-worth in children. In N. Eisenberg (Ed.), *Contemporary topics in developmental psychology* (pp. 219–242). New York: Wiley.

Harter, S. (1990). Causes, correlates, and the functional role of global self-worth: A life-span perspective. In J. Kolligian & R. Sternberg (Eds.), *Perceptions of competence and incompetence across the life-span* (pp. 67–98). New Haven, CT: Yale University Press.

Harter, S. (1998). The effects of child abuse on the self-system. In B. B. R. Rossman & M. S. Rosenberg (Eds.), *Multiple victimization of children: Conceptual, developmental, research, and treatment issues* (pp. 147–170). New York: Haworth Press.

Harter, S. (1999). *The construction of the self: A developmental perspective.* New York: Guilford Press.

Held, B. S. (1995). *Back to reality: A critique of postmodern theory in psychotherapy.* New York: Norton.

Herman, J. L. (1981). *Father–daughter incest.* Cambridge, MA: Harvard University Press.

Herman, J. L. (1992). *Trauma and recovery.* New York: Basic Books.

Hildebrand, J. (1988). The use of groupwork in treating child sexual abuse. In A. Bentovim, A. Elton, J. Hildebrand, M. Tranter, & E. Vizard (Eds.), *Child sexual abuse within the family* (pp. 205–237). London: Wright.

Hoffman, L. (1985). Beyond power and control: Toward a "second order" family systems therapy. *Family Systems Medicine, 3,* 381–396.

Hoffman, L. (1990). Constructing realities: An art of lenses. *Family Process, 29,* 1–12.

Howes, P. W., Ciccehetti, D., Toth, S. L., & Rogosch, F. (2000). Affective, organizational, and relational characteristics of maltreating families: A systems perspective. *Journal of Family Psychology, 14*, 95–110.

Hunter, W. M., Coulter, M. L., Runyan, D. K., & Everson, M. D. (1990). Determinants of placement for sexually abused children. *Child Abuse and Neglect, 14*, 407–418.

Hunter, J., Goodwin, D.W., & Wilson, R. J. (1992). Attributions of blame in child sexual abuse victims: An analysis of age and gender influences. *Journal of Child Sexual Abuse, 1*, 75–90.

Imber-Black, E. (1988). *Families and larger systems: A family therapist's guide through the labyrinth.* New York: Guilford Press.

James, K., & MacKinnon, L. (1990). The "incestuous" family revisited: A critical analysis of family therapy myths. *Journal of Marital and Family Therapy, 16*, 71–88.

Jenkins, A. (1990). *Invitations to responsibility: The therapeutic engagement of men who are violent and abusive.* Adelaide, Australia: Dulwich Centre Publications.

Johnson, T. C. (1993). Group therapy. In E. Gil & T. C. Johnson (Eds.), *Sexualized children: Assessment and treatment of sexualized children and children who molest* (pp. 211–273). Rockville, MD: Launch Press.

Johnson, T. C., & Feldmeth, J. R. (1993). Sexual behaviors: A continuum. In E. Gil & T. C. Johnson (Eds.), *Sexualized children: Assessment and treatment of sexualized children and children who molest* (pp. 41–52). Rockville, MD: Launch Press.

Jordan, J., Kaplan, A., Miller, J. B., Stiver, I., & Surrey, J. (1991). *Women's growth in connection: Writings from the Stone Center.* New York: Guilford Press.

Joyce, P. A. (1997). Mothers of sexually abused children and the concept of collusion: A literature review. *Journal of Child Sexual Abuse, 6*, 75–92.

Kaslow, F. W. (Ed.). (1996). *Handbook of relational diagnosis and dysfunctional family patterns.* New York: Wiley.

Kendall-Tackett, K. A., Williams, L. M., & Finkelhor, D. (1993). Impact of sexual abuse on children: A review and synthesis of recent empirical studies. *Psychological Bulletin, 113*, 164–180.

Kerr, M., & Bowen, M. (1988). *Family evaluation.* New York: Norton.

Ketring, S. A., & Feinhauer, L. L. (1999). Perpetrator–victim relationship: Long-term effects of sexual abuse for men and women. *American Journal of Family Therapy, 27*, 109–120.

Knutson, J. F. (1995). Psychological characteristics of maltreated children: Putative risk factors and consequences. *Annual Review of Psychology, 46*, 401–431.

Lawson, L., & Chaffin, M. (1992). False negatives in sexual abuse disclosure interviews: Incidence and influence of caretakers' belief in abuse in cases of accidental abuse discovery by diagnosis of STD. *Journal of Interpersonal Violence, 7*, 532–542.

Lebow, J. (1997). The integrative revolution in couple and family therapy. *Family Process, 36*, 1–17.

Levitt, C. J., Owen, G., & Truchsess, J. (1991). Families after sexual abuse: What helps? What is needed? In M. Q. Patton (Ed.), *Family sexual abuse: Frontline research and evaluation* (pp. 39–56). Newbury Park, CA: Sage.

Libow, J. A., Raskin, P. A., & Caust, B. L. (1982). Feminist and family systems therapy: Are they irreconcilable? *American Journal of Family Therapy, 10*, 3–12.

Loftus, E. F., & Ketcham, K. (1994). *The myth of repressed memory.* New York: St. Martin's Press.

Longo, R. F., Bays, L., & Bear, E. (1996). *Empathy and compassionate action: Issues and exercises: A workbook for clients in treatment.* Brandon, VT: Safer Society Press.

Luthar, S. S., & Zigler, E. (1991). Vulnerability and competence: A review of research on resilience in childhood. *American Journal of Orthopsychiatry, 61*, 6–22.

Madanes, C. (1990). *Sex, love, and violence: Strategies for transformation.* New York: Norton.

Maletzky, B. M. (1991). *Treating the sexual offender.* Thousand Oaks, CA: Sage.

Mandell, J. G., Damon, L., Castaldo, P., Tauber, E., Monise, L., & Larsen, N. (1989). *Group treatment of sexually abused children.* New York: Guilford Press.

Marshall, W. L., Laws, D. R., & Barbaree, H. E. (Eds.). (1990). *Handbook of sexual assault: Issues, theories, and treatment of the offender.* New York: Plenum.

McNamee, S., & Gergen, K. (Eds.). (1992). *Therapy as social construction.* London: Sage.

McNay, L. (1992). *Foucault and feminism: Power, gender, and the self.* Boston: Northeastern University Press.

Mead, G. H. (1934). *Mind, self, and society.* Chicago: University of Chicago Press.

Miller, R., & Dwyer, J. (1997). Reclaiming the mother–daughter relationship after sexual abuse. *Australian and New Zealand Journal of Family Therapy, 18*, 194–202.

Minuchin, P., Colapinto, J., & Minuchin, S. (1998). *Working with families of the poor.* New York: Guilford Press.

Mrazek, P. B., & Bentovim, A. (1981). Incest and the dysfunctional family system. In P. B. Mrazek & C. H. Kempe (Eds.), *Sexually abused children and their families* (pp. 167–178). Oxford, England: Pergamon Press.

Murphy, W. D., & Smith, T. A. (1996). Sex offenders against children. In J. Briere, L. Berliner, J. A. Bulkley, C. Jenny, & T. Reid (Eds.), *The APSAC handbook on child maltreatment* (pp. 175–191). Thousand Oaks, CA: Sage.

National Clearinghouse on Child Abuse and Neglect Information. (1996). *Child abuse and neglect fact sheet.* Washington, DC: Author.

Nelki, J. S., & Walters, J. (1989). A group for sexually abused young children: Unravelling the web. *Child Abuse and Neglect, 13*, 369–377.

Norcross, J. C., & Newman, C. F. (1992). Psychotherapy integration: Setting the context. In J. C. Norcross & M. R. Goldfried (Eds.), *Handbook of psychotherapy integration* (pp. 3–45). New York: Basic Books.

Paré, D. A. (1995). Of families and other cultures: The shifting paradigm of family therapy. *Family Process, 34,* 1–19.

Paré, D. A. (1996). Culture and meaning: Expanding the metaphorical repertoire of family therapy. *Family Process, 35,* 21–42.

Parker, H., & Parker, S. (1986). Father–daughter sexual abuse: An emerging perspective. *American Journal of Orthopsychiatry, 56,* 531–549.

Peck, J. S., Sheinberg, M., & Akamatsu, N. N. (1995). Forming a consortium: A design for interagency collaboration in the delivery of service following the disclosure of incest. *Family Process, 34,* 287–302.

Peters, S. D. (1988). Child abuse and later psychological problems. In G. E. Wyatt & G. J. Powell (Eds.), *Lasting effects on child sexual abuse* (pp. 101–118). Newbury Park, CA: Sage.

Peters, S. D., Wyatt, G. E., & Finkelhor, D. (1986). Prevalence. In D. Finkelhor & Associates, *A sourcebook on child sexual abuse* (pp. 15–59). Newbury Park, CA: Sage.

Prentky, R. A. (1998). *Juvenile Risk Assessment Scale.* Unpublished scale, Boston, MA.

Reiss, D. (1981). *The family's construction of reality.* Cambridge, MA: Harvard University Press.

Russell, D. E. (1983). The incidence and prevalence of intrafamilial and extrafamilial sexual abuse of female children. *Child Abuse and Neglect, 7,* 133–146.

Russell, D. E. (1984). The prevalence and seriousness of incestuous abuse: Stepfathers versus biological fathers. *Child Abuse and Neglect, 8,* 15–22.

Ryan, G., & Lane, S. (Eds.). (1997). *Juvenile sexual offending: Causes, consequences, and correction* (2nd ed.). San Francisco: Jossey-Bass.

Salter, A. C. (1988). *Treating child sex offenders and victims: A practical guide.* Newbury Park, CA: Sage.

Schwartz, B. K., & Cellini, H. R. (Eds.). (1995). *The sex offender: Corrections, treatment, and legal practice.* Kingston, NJ: Civic Research Institute.

Sedlak, A. J., & Broadhurst, D. D. (1996). *Third national incidence study of child abuse and neglect: Final report.* Washington, DC: National Center on Child Abuse and Neglect, Department of Health and Human Services.

Sgroi, S. M. (1982). *Handbook of clinical intervention in child sexual abuse.* Lexington, MA: Lexington Books.

Sheinberg, M. (1992). Navigating treatment impasses at the disclosure of incest: Combining ideas from feminism and social constructionism. *Family Process, 31,* 201–216.

Sheinberg, M., True, F., & Fraenkel, P. (1994). Treating the sexually abused child: A recursive, multimodal program. *Family Process, 33,* 263–276.

Sheinberg, M., & Penn, P. (1991). Gender dilemmas, gender questions and the gender mantra. *Journal of Marital and Family Therapy, 17,* 33–44.

Sorensen, T., & Snow, B. (1991). How children tell: The process of disclosure in child sexual abuse. *Child Welfare League of America, 70*, 3–15.

Spaccarelli, S. (1994). Stress, appraisal, and coping in child sexual abuse: A theoretical and empirical review. *Psychological Bulletin, 116*, 11–23.

Spaccarelli, S., & Kim, S. (1995). Resilience criteria and factors associated with resilience in sexually abused girls. *Child Abuse and Neglect, 19*, 1171–1182.

Trepper, T. S., & Barrett, M. J. (1989). *Systemic treatment of incest: A therapeutic handbook.* New York: Brunner/Mazel.

Trepper, T. S., & Neidner, D. M. (1996). Intrafamily child sexual abuse. In F. W. Kaslow (Ed.), *Handbook of relational diagnosis and dysfunctional family patterns* (pp. 394–406). New York: Wiley.

U.S. Department of Health and Human Services, National Center on Child Abuse and Neglect. (1996). *Child maltreatment 1994: Reports from the states to the National Center on Child Abuse and Neglect.* Washington, DC: U.S. Government Printing Office.

van der Kolk, B. A., McFarlane, A. C., & van der Hart, O. (1996). A general approach to treatment of posttraumatic stress disorder. In B. A. van der Kolk, A. C. McFarlane, & L. Weisaeth (Eds.), *Traumatic stress: The effects of overwhelming experience on mind, body, and society* (pp. 417–440). New York: Guilford Press.

van der Kolk, B. A., McFarlane, A. C., & Weisaeth, L. (1996). *Traumatic stress: The effects of overwhelming experience on mind, body, and society.* New York: Guilford Press.

Walsh, F. (1998). *Strengthening family resilience.* New York: Guilford Press.

Walley, M. (1993). Empathy and prosocial development. In K. N. Bwivedi (Ed.), *Group work with children and adolescents: A handbook* (pp. 78–98). London: Jessica Kingsley.

White, M. (1992). Deconstruction and therapy. In D. Epston & M. White (Eds.), *Experience, contradiction, narrative, and imagination: Selected papers of David Epston and Michael White* (pp. 109–151). Adelaide, South Australia: Dulwich Centre Publications.

White, M., & Epston, D. (1990). *Narrative means to therapeutic ends.* New York: Norton.

Wiese, D., & Daro, D. (1995). *Current trends in child abuse reporting and fatalities: The results of the 1994 annual fifty state survey.* Chicago: National Committee to Prevent Child Abuse.

Williams, L. (1994). Recall of childhood trauma: A prospective study of women's memories of child sexual abuse. *Journal of Consulting and Clinical Psychology, 62*, 1167–1176.

Williams, L. M., & Finkelhor, D. (1995). Paternal caregiving and incest: Test of a biosocial model. *American Journal of Orthopsychiatry, 65*, 101–113.

Wyatt, G. E., & Mickey, M. R. (1988). The support by parents and others as it mediates the effects of child sexual abuse: An exploratory study. In G. E. Wyatt

& G. J. Powell (Eds.), *Lasting effects of child sexual abuse* (pp. 211–226). Newbury Park, CA: Sage.

Yapko, M. (1994). *Suggestions of abuse: True and false memories of childhood sexual trauma.* New York: Simon & Schuster.

Zimmerman, J. L., & Dickerson, V. C. (1994). Using a narrative metaphor: Implications for theory and clinical practice. *Family Process, 33,* 233–245.

Index